W9-APM-101

Working the Web:
A Guide for Nurses

Julie B. Bliss, Ed.D., M.Ed., M.A.
Associate Professor of Nursing
College of Science and Health
William Paterson University
Wayne, New Jersey

Sandra DeYoung, Ed.D., M.Ed., M.A.
Associate Dean and Professor of Nursing
College of Science and Health
William Paterson University
Wayne, New Jersey

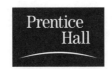

Prentice
Hall

Upper Saddle River, New Jersey 07458

Library of Congress Cataloging-in-Publication Data
Bliss, Julie B.
    Working the web: a guide for nurses / Julie B. Bliss, Sandra De Young.
      p.; cm.
    Includes index.
    ISBN 0-13-061788-1
    1. Nursing—Computer network resource.   2. Web site—Ratings. I. De Young, Sandra.
    II. Title.
    [DNLM: 1. Internet—Nurses' Instruction. WY 26.5 B649w 2002]
    RT50.5 .B553 2002
    025.06´61073—dc21

                                                  2001036603

Publisher: Julie Alexander
Executive Editor: Maura Connor
Director of Production and Manufacturing: Bruce Johnson
Managing Production Editor: Patrick Walsh
Manufacturing Buyer: Pat Brown
Production Liaison: Julie Li
Production Editor: Karen Fortgang, *bookworks*
Creative Director: Cheryl Asherman
Cover Design Coordinator: Maria Guglielmo
Marketing Manager: Nicole Benson
Media Development Editor: Sarah Hayday
Editorial Assistant: Beth Ann Romph
Composition: Rainbow Graphics
Printing and Binding: Banta Group/Eden Prairie

Pearson Education LTD.
Pearson Education Australia PTY, Limited
Pearson Education Singapore, Pte. Ltd
Pearson Education North Asia Ltd
Pearson Education Canada, Ltd.
Pearson Educación de Mexico, S.A. de C.V.
Pearson Education–Japan
Pearson Education Malaysia, Pte. Ltd
Pearson Education, Upper Saddle River, New Jersey

Copyright © 2002 by Pearson Education, Inc., Upper Saddle River, New Jersey 07458. All
rights reserved. Printed in the United States of America. This publication is protected by Copyright and permission should be obtained from the publisher prior to any prohibited reproduction,
storage in a retrieval system, or transmission in any form or by any means, electronic, mechani-
cal, photocopying, recording, or likewise. For information regarding permission(s), write to:
Rights and Permissions Department.

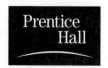

10 9 8 7 6 5 4 3 2 1
ISBN 0-13-061788-1

Contents

*To my father, Woodrow P. Beshore, who encouraged me
to embrace and not fear the power of machines . . .*

Julie Beshore Bliss

*To my brother, Bruce DeYoung, who taught me how to turn
on my computer, and so much more . . .*

Sandra DeYoung

Preface

Many of us began using the Internet in a hit-or-miss, trial-and-error fashion. If we were lucky, eventually we found what we were looking for. However, when you are using the Internet for professional purposes, a systematic, informed approach is much more efficient and will produce quality information that you can use to benefit yourself, your colleagues, and your patients.

This book is designed to be a useful manual for the novice or intermediate-level Internet user. The first five chapters of this book contain the background information needed to get you up-to-speed quickly. We then progress to more advanced information on searching the Web and protecting your privacy.

Chapter 1 describes the Internet and the equipment and resources needed to access it. Means of connecting to the Internet are explained, as is the logic of Web site addresses.

Chapter 2 covers Internet applications, including e-mail, e-mail etiquette, and mailbox use. Also covered are listservs and their use, newsgroups, and chat rooms.

Chapter 3 explores World Wide Web search techniques. Search engines and metasearch engines are defined, and examples are given. Basic and advanced search techniques using Boolean logic are explained.

Chapter 4 encompasses means by which you can evaluate the quality and usefulness of Web sites. This will help you decide which Web sites you can have faith in. Privacy issues with Internet use are discussed.

Chapter 5 deals with continuing education and college courses that can be found online. Criteria for evaluating the courses are included, as well as criteria for helping you decide if online learning is for you.

Chapter 6 encompasses the rest of the book, and it contains over 300 Web sites that we believe are potentially useful to nursing students and practicing nurses. The sites are categorized by functional unit, such as Anatomy and Physiology, Care Plans, Evidence-Based Practice, History of Nursing, Medication Calculation, Orthopedics, Pain, and Women's Health. Each Web site has been evaluated by us as to clarity of purpose, currency, credibility, content accuracy, and design, and each site has been given a rating from * (poor) to ***** (excellent). Our annotations of the sites indicate the most useful nuggets of information that can be found there. For additional resources and exercises, go to the free Companion Website accompanying this book at www.prenhall.com/bliss.

We believe you will find this book helpful as you seek to use the incredible resources found on the Internet. We hope you will also find it enjoyable. Have fun!

Julie Bliss

Sandra DeYoung

Reviewers

Randy De Kler, Ph.D., M.S.
Georgia State University
Atlanta, GA

Elizabeth Elkind, R.N.C., M.S.N., M.B.A.
Thomas Jefferson University
Philadelphia, PA

Joan Fleitas, Ed.D.
Fairfield University
Fairfield, CT

Peggy L. Hawkins, R.N., Ph.D.
College of Saint Mary
Omaha, NE

Getting Started

At the beginning of the Second Millennium we are fortunate to have a fairly direct path to getting started using the Internet. All we need is the right equipment, a desire to learn, and time to work the Web. This is simple for us, but those who have gone before have struggled, even competed, to develop pathways that facilitate the ease of use that is currently available. A few facts related to these developments follow.

HOW THE WORLD WIDE WEB BEGAN

Although the United States is generally thought to be the creator of the Internet, many think tanks and research institutions around the world contributed to its development. In the late 1950s, the Department of Defense funded a project, known as the DOD Advanced Research Projects Agency (DARPA), to link military and government institutions in the event of a military or natural disaster; its purpose was to create a data communication system.

In 1968, three diverse groups, who were working on using data packets to transmit information, met to develop a data network. This group included the RAND corporation, DARPA, and the National Physical Laboratory (NPL) in Middlesex, England (Zakon, 2000). Their solution to this communication problem was a "fancy telephone system." No voice was involved, but connections were the key. Electronic packets of data were sent from one location to another, but rather than traveling directly they were routed to travel along different paths and to come together at the destination. They traveled as fast as electricity. This project developed into the Advanced Research Project Association Network

(ARPANET), a communication network that eventually became known as the Web (as in spider web).

The Web expanded with the addition of research universities, who wanted to speed up the development of new knowledge by sharing information faster than the print medium. To facilitate this, in the early 1980s the National Science Foundation funded the establishment of several supercomputer centers that connected to the ARPANET Communication Web. These centers were established at the University of California–Los Angeles (UCLA), Carnegie-Mellon University (CMU), the Massachusetts Institute of Technology (MIT), and the University of Illinois. Scientists working on the project envisioned many potential users of this communication network and saw the need to develop site names for the users, in addition to the numbers used for their addresses. Categories, or domains, for usage were determined to be in six areas: military, education, government, nonprofit organizations, commercial, and computer Internet concerns. These domains were identified by a three-letter designation, called extensions, within the site address as follows: .mil, .edu, .gov, .org, .com, and .net., respectively.

The first Internet addresses were registered in 1984. The Internet Corporation for Assigned Names and Numbers (ICANN) is currently responsible for domain name system management. In November 2000 they voted to expand the top level domains to include: .biz, .info, .name, .pro, .museum, .aero, and .coop. These will become available to businesses and consumers by mid-2001 (Eric Lai, Reuters, © 2000 News24). Internet sites may also have a country code. A list of the country codes can be found at *www.norid.no/domreg.html.*

Early developers of the Internet used protocols, or rules, to standardize the transmission of data. They created protocols for e-mail and FTP (File Transfer Protocol) files, discussion boards, and eventually HTML (Hypertext Markup Language) files. Each of these operations has its own rules for data exchange.

Although originally only large mainframe computers could exchange data, today anyone can access data using personal computers—some small enough to be handheld!

In order to "Work the Web," you need a personal computer (hardware), an Internet browser (software program), and a connection to the Internet Service Provider (ISP) of your choice. The earliest proprietary ISPs were AOL, CompuServe, and Prodigy; today there are many more providers from which to choose.

CHOOSING A COMPUTER

What type of computer do I really need to "Work the Web"? If you are planning to use your information for further reference or for sharing information with clients, you need a computer that is capable of doing several things with the information accessed on the Web. This is called multitasking, and requires software that facilitates word processing, spreadsheet functions, and desktop publishing, and includes a music/video player and an e-mail utility. Would a Web TV be all right? No, because Web TV does not have these multitasking capabilities.

How much computer should I buy? You will probably be very happy with a computer that has about half the processing power of the current top-of-the-line computer. That is, if the current top-of-the-line computer advertised is 1.2 GHz, then you would be happy surfing the Web with a computer with 600 MHz processing speed. You can go high-end with lots of bells and whistles or you can go low end with just the basics. Consult an established computer dealer for advice on making these choices. Whatever you decide, do not compromise on screen size. If you have any intentions of "Working the Web" either for your own enjoyment or employment, or for your patients, you will want to have at least a 17-inch monitor. Many Internet pages will require that you use a horizontal scroll bar to see the whole page, and this process is cumbersome on a 14-inch screen. Table 1–1 offers suggestions gleaned from current major computer companies regarding basic components and their relative prices as of this writing.

SELECTING A BROWSER

A browser is a computer application that allows users to view Web sites that may contain text, sound, images, and/or video. This is enabled using a system of coding known as hypertext markup language (HTML) that all browsers read and then display on your monitor/cathode ray tube (CRT)/screen. There are two major browsers in use in the United States today: Microsoft Internet Explorer and Netscape Navigator. Other browsers are available, for example, Opera, Neoplanet, and Ariadna developed in Germany, Norway, and Russia, respectively. These are used primarily in Europe. See *www.cnet.com/internet/0-3773.html* for more information.

Table 1-1	Computer Components Needed to Get Started	
	Minimum Needed	**Maximum Wanted**
Processor	600 MHz	1.5 GHz
RAM	64 Mb	256 Mb
Hard drive	5 Gb	80 Gb
Mouse	Two-button ball mouse	Optical wheel mouse
CD	24 X max	8x/4x/32x CD-RW, 2nd bay
Monitor	14″ monitor	19″ monitor
Floppy drive	3.5″ floppy drive	3.5″ floppy drive
Sound card	Wavetable sound card	ISA wavetable sound card
Speakers	Integrated speakers	Surround sound speakers, subwoofer
Price	$600	$3,000

CONNECTING TO AN INTERNET SERVICE PROVIDER (ISP)

Most readers of this book already have access to a computer with a connection to the Internet either at home, a library, a cyber café, or school. However, if you are planning to buy a computer to access the Web, consider the following. First, the most important component to "working the web" and enjoying the experience is your connection speed. The faster your connection, the faster the pages you want to view will appear. If you are connecting from home, currently the least expensive, most prevalent (available) connection is through a telephone modem.

The modem (<u>mo</u>dulator–<u>dem</u>odulator) is the equipment that converts your text, graphics, or sound into electronic packets to travel the Internet and vice versa: to translate the electronic packets received by your computer into their intended message (text, graphics, and sound). The more complex the message, the greater the amount of electronic data needed to display the message as intended. The cliché "a picture is worth a thousand words" is validated in Internet processes. That is, text is very simple to translate into code and is quickly downloaded to your computer, but where pictures, graphics, sound, color, and/or movement are included, the coding becomes complex and requires a lot more time to transmit as intended. Of course we like pictures and sound and movement. So, to enjoy "working the web" we need to be able to access a lot of data (information packets) quickly.

Currently, the speeds of dial-up telephone modems are either 28.8 kbps or 56.6 kbps (kilobits per second). This translates into approximately 1024×28.8 typed letters (29491.2 letters) per second, because a bit (binary digit) is either a 0 or 1. Internet connections are very inexpensive, from no cost to $25 per month plus the cost of the telephone call to your ISP. Most ISP connections are local numbers, but if you have to call long distance, the costs can increase rapidly. Of course you can't talk on the telephone while you are on the Internet so you may want to install a second telephone line. You may also find that you have to wait to get connected because you are getting a busy signal at your ISP. If there are a lot of members on the same dial-up node, you may get a busy signal or be "thrown-off," or "timed out," if you are not constantly exchanging data.

After telephone modem connections came broadband connections, which allow a large amount of data to be transmitted quickly. The most common type available to the public is the Digital Subscriber Line (DSL). There are several variations on the type and speed of this category of connection. Generally, telephone companies provide DSLs. One drawback is that the distance from the connection affects the speed of the data transfer; thus, they are not recommended for anyone more than 20,000 feet (about 5 miles) from the central location of the company. On the plus side, they are relatively troublefree, almost never lose their connections, and do not require a separate telephone line. These connections require a modem but once connected they are always on, representing a significant risk to your privacy. The selection of a synchronous or asynchronous connection may depend on your pocketbook. A synchronous connection is one where the sending and receiving speed is the same. An asynchronous connection (by far the most common) has a faster receiving or downloading speed than sending or upstream speed. Faster is more expensive. The speeds vary from 16 kbps upstream to 9 Mbps downstream (16,384 to 6,291,456 bits per second). Generally the most important speed is the download rate, unless you are uploading large files (Bass, 2000).

A third Internet connection possibility is the cable modems, which are becoming increasingly common. If you receive your television signal via a cable, then you may be able to also connect to the Internet via the same cable with a modem. The speed is comparable to the closest DSL connections, averaging 1 Mbps upstream to 4 Mbps downloading. This translates to 1 to 4 million bps. Like the DSL, most cable modems have faster download speeds than upstream speeds. There is no waiting to check a password or obtain an available line. The downside is that because the connection is always on, you are very vulnerable to hackers and snoopers. For some, television cable connections are unreliable; hence access to the Internet will also be lost.

One current advertising campaign suggests that we really can't live without a wireless modem connection to the Internet. This is a nice idea whose technology is still being developed. Not unlike the cell phone phenomenon, wireless connections are great if you are in receiving range of a transmitter, but if you are in a "dead spot" you are out of luck. Wireless connections used to be relatively slow, but new high-speed standards of 11 Mbps are making this option increasingly attractive.

Satellite connections to the Internet are also on the horizon. Although they are currently available for both upstream and downloading, some still require a dial-up connection to upload data. The speed for upstream may be as low as 28.8 kbps and download as fast as 500 kbps. Therefore the efficiency is about half that of a DSL or cable connection. Also, be sure you do not have a large tree near your dish that blocks access to the desired satellite.

Your ability to work the Web primarily depends on your connection to the Internet and *not* your processing power. With expensive computers, there may be enhancement of quality but generally not of quantity or access. Therefore, we recommend that you buy or find the fastest broadband connection within your means, rather than the most expensive computer available.

REFERENCES

Bass, S. (2000). High speed survival guide. *PC World, 18*(8), 145–57.

FNC Resolution: Definition of Internet 10/24/95 (1995). Washington, DC: Federal Networking Council. Retrieved December 18, 2000, from the World Wide Web: *www.fnc.gov/Internet_res.html*

Lai, E. Seven new domains. Reuters (November 11, 2000). Retrieved December 18, 2000, from the World Wide Web: *news.24.com/News24/Technology/Infotech/0,1113,2-13-45_941655,00.html*

Spanbauer, S. (2001). Fast-access face off. *PC World, 19*(1), 94–97.

Utility Guide Broadband Speed Chart. Retrieved December 19, 2000, from the World Wide Web: *www.utilityguide.com/internet. cfm?b= speed_chart2000*

Zakon, R. H. (November 2000). *Hobbes' Internet Timeline v5.2.* Retrieved December 18, 2000, from the World Wide Web: *www.isoc.org/guest/zakon/Internet/History/HIT.html*

2

Using the World Wide Web

Using the World Wide Web (WWW) has been made very simple. With most connections to the Internet (see Chapter 1) you begin by logging on. Logging on requires that you enter a username and password. Everyone has a name/number or identifier in cyberspace. You may use your real name, an alias, or a code. This is needed so that your requests for information can be returned to you and your e-mail can be responded to. If your anonymity is important, you will need to use an anonymous re-mailer application (downloadable from the Internet). But primarily you do have an identity. No one is not identified. If you are in a public computer laboratory, your computer has an identity on the Internet. This chapter will discuss several protocols that enable data transfer and some suggestions for using them. E-mail is a "killer application" that established the indispensability of the Internet. People found the application useful, easy to use, and faster than other types of communication, except for the telephone. Thus it made work and play more efficient. E-mail has become ubiquitous, perhaps not as much as the telephone or television at this writing, but it surely will in the near future. Other application protocols discussed in this chapter include listservs, bulletin boards, newsgroups, and chat rooms. Searching the Internet as an application follows with its own chapter.

E-MAIL

Electronic mail is the most used Internet application. It preceded surfing the Web, and it requires less connection speed, no browser, and a minimum of processing power. E-mail is like the postal service, except it travels in MHz time rather than days or weeks, and it can only be delivered to a cyber address. Geographic locations are immaterial. It is delivered only to Internet mailboxes, sometimes called screen names. It arrives nearly instantaneously, depending on the speed of your connection and to some extent the volume of traffic on the local networks. Mail can get lost but this is a rare event. The mail stays on your electronic Internet host (ISP) server until you download the messages. Hence, e-mail is considered an asynchronous communication tool. Unlike the telephone, both parties do not have to be home or on the Internet to receive or send e-mail. In addition, e-mail can be sent at anytime without waking the recipient. Your recipients will open their mail at their own convenience.

Applications that handle e-mail vary widely in appearance and functionality. Some allow only text and keyboard commands, while others support HTML (the language of the Internet), sound, graphics, file attachments, and are GUI (graphical user interface) compliant. The speed of the transmission is not affected by the type of application but by the size of the message. Graphics and sound files require a lot of information to display and are therefore large files.

E-mail is not secure. This means unintended audiences can access your mail while it is in route to its destination—like eavesdropping on a telephone conversation. This may be accidental, innocent, purposeful (on the job), or malicious. Some have said that nothing should be put in an e-mail that you would not put on a post card. E-mail can be protected via encryption but this is usually not done unless sensitive information (like a credit card number) is being transmitted. This technology may soon be used for personal health care information providers as they offer Web-based patient access to their health records (a likely scenario as the 1996 Kennedy–Kassenbaum Act becomes law).

In addition to the convenience of fast communication, e-mail also makes us vulnerable to computer viruses or other unfriendly miseries. To this we recommend that you install a virus protector (software program) on your computer. This program will scan all of your files for currently known viruses before you open them. And when sending e-mail use the text only or text-rich format and not HTML code. If you code your messages in HTML, they look colorful and fancy but they also allow troubling programs to be imbedded in the message without your knowledge. If someone sends you an HTML or executable file (has an .exe extension) do not open it directly but rather download it to a disk. Then open the file from your disk. Your resident virus protection program will intercept any corrupting or unfriendly hidden applications.

If you do not already have an e-mail account, get one. It will change your way of communicating, for the better. And you may wonder how you ever got along without it.

E-MAIL ETIQUETTE

The following guidelines will help you be a responsible user.

1. Get the right (correct) address of the person to whom you are sending your message. Guessing at an address may send your message to the wrong person.
2. Put a topic in the subject section of the e-mail header. Sending a blank subject e-mail may mean your message is automatically deleted by the reader who thinks it must not be important.
3. Do not just start your message. Greet your intended audience, for example, "Hi Rita." This is both courteous and is a check that the correct person has received your message.
4. Keep your messages short. A 15-page message is not fun to read and may not be given much priority, unless of course it is a required writing assignment for a course you are taking. (In this case it is better to send the assignment as an attachment.)
5. Respond to e-mails in a timely manner. Set up a personal schedule for checking your e-mail, either daily or on a certain day of the week. Messages can be marked as important so that the recipient is flagged when the message arrives. Most messages are *not* high priorities.

As you become e-mail proficient you will want to "tidy your mailbox." Typically there is an Inbox (where messages arrive); an Outbox, or Sent, mail folder (where copies of all your sent messages are kept); and a Delete box (messages you meant to delete). You will want to organize your files or mailboxes. Following are some ideas.

• Create folders in your Inbox to keep messages that you have read but want to save for reference (you do not have to print out the messages). For example, you may want a folder for work, relatives, research, and/or jokes/humor. You can make subfolders in these folders; for example, in your research folder you could have a pilot study file, references file, forms file, and so on.

- Go to your Sent mailbox about once a week and delete any messages that you do not need to keep.
- Go to your Deleted mailbox and, after reviewing the items and determining that you do not want them, delete them or empty the deleted items box (folder).

Now you are organized!

LISTSERVS

The concept of the listserv is a group e-mail system. Individuals subscribe to a group. They choose to join because of an interest in the acknowledged topic to be discussed on the listserv. Some listservs are moderated and some are not; some have an open membership and some require permission to join. There are hundreds or perhaps thousands of health-related listservs. Some are for professionals; some are for patients, for students, or for families. It is often difficult to tell the nature of a listserv until you join.

Every listserv has two addresses. **This is important.** To join a listserv you must send a message to the administrative address. This is the address of the computer/server, where the program lives or resides. The second address is the list address where messages are sent for distribution to the subscribers. An example of an administrative address is *listserv@list.university.edu.* An example of a list address is *GradNurse@list.university.edu.* In these examples, *listserv/GradNurse* is the mailbox where the message is processed; @ is the symbol used only in e-mail that separates the mailbox name from the list address; *list* is the name of the server; *university* is where the server resides; and *edu* is the domain of the listserv location.

To join a listserv you must send a command to the administrative address. The computer/listserv application understands only specific commands (spelled correctly). Usually the subject area is left blank. In the body of the message, type the designated command to subscribe or join (depending on the directions of the list program/application) followed by the name of the list that you wish to join. Many list managers also request the name of the person requesting to join. Thus, a request to join our GradNurse mailing list above would require the following command to the Administrative address: subscribe GradNurse Sally Student. A welcome message is returned to Sally Student at her e-mail address when she is successful. You should save the welcome message. It will tell you how to remove your name from the mailing list or perform various other tasks such as temporarily holding your mail or grouping your mail to receive only one group of messages per day. Some listservs put the unsubscribe directions at the end of every message for easy reference.

To participate in the discussion, you will need to use the list address. In the example above, send a message to *GradNurse@list.university.edu*; indicate the topic of your message in the Subject area; type your message and send it. You may also only "lurk," that is, just read the messages others have posted on the listserv. You can learn a lot on an electronic mailing list.

NEWSGROUPS

Newsgroups use an Internet protocol, which also runs on servers (computers), and act as managers of messages posted by anyone sending a message to that address. Newsgroups are like listservs in that they typically use the e-mail system of message sharing, are asynchronous, and typically are focused on a narrow content area. However, unlike listservs, you do not have to "belong" to participate. Newsgroups are not really "news" but more like a bulletin board where you can ask a question or ask for advice or share an experience with anyone who signs on to your group (newsgroup). There are thousands of newsgroups but few nursing-relevant sites. Newsgroups are heavily used outside the United States.

CHAT ROOMS

Chat rooms are also known as IRCs (Internet Relay Chat). These are computer applications that allow synchronous communication. This is very much like talking on the telephone but typically you see only the typed messages. The advantage is the real-time exchange of information. A disadvantage is that the fastest typist often monopolizes the so-called conversation. Adolescents, not surprisingly, love this application of the Internet; the Instant Message application developed by AOL (America On Line) is extremely popular with the junior high through college crowd. Telephone calls via the Internet are a form of IRC; these can include voice (sound card and microphone) and pictures (video camera). Nurses are beginning to use IRCs to facilitate support groups for specific illnesses. Thus, IRCs may be moderated, that is, an expert is on hand to give advice, or may be unmoderated so that individuals may communicate with anyone who signs into the "room." Typically less than 10 people are recommended. It is harder to "lurk" on IRCs because all of the signed on participants' usernames are listed at all times.

There are many applications available on the Internet. E-mail has revolutionized communication, especially since the late 1990s, and numerous applications continue to develop that capitalized on the world's fascination with asynchronous and synchronous electronic communication. Soon the videophone will not seem outrageous. We have loved sending and receiving our pictures using still and video technology. Try your hand at a listserv or a newsgroup. Sign into a health-related chat. It is fun, interesting, and stimulating to converse with an unknown but perhaps like-minded individual.

3

Searching the World Wide Web

You have probably heard of people "surfing" the World Wide Web (WWW). This phrase usually means that people just meander around the Web, following one link to another, pausing at what interests them. When you surf the ocean you stay on the surface of the water for the most part; when you "surf" the Web, you stay on the surface of all the good information that exists on a topic. To dive deeper into a topic, or to broaden your coverage of it, you will want to search the Web in a systematic way.

SEARCH TOOLS

Search tools (often called search engines) were developed to help people look for specific topics on the Web. The WWW consists of more than a billion pages and documents. In fact, growth of the Web is so rapid that no one knows for sure just how large the number is. Because it is so large, if you want to save time and search efficiently, you'll want to use a search tool. There are many from which to choose (see Table 3–1).

Every search tool compiles a database of Internet sites, including WWW sites. The size of the database in each search tool varies. The search tool needs not only a database, but also an engine, which is a computer program that uses rules of logic to actually search the database (Sparks & Rizzolo, 1998). The search engine then indexes Web pages and gives the URL (uniform resource locator or address) for each page.

According to a 1998 study, the best search engines at that time covered about one-third of the Web, while many covered significantly less (Lawrence & Giles, 1998). The publication of these

Table 3–1 Popular Search Engines	
Search Engine	**URL**
AltaVista	*www.altavista.com*
FAST	*www.alltheweb.com*
Hotbot	*hotbot.lycos.com*
MSN	*msn.com*
Netscape	*netscape.com*
Northernlight	*northernlight.com*
Oingo	*www.oingo.com*
WebCrawler	*www.webcrawler.com*
Yahoo!	*www.yahoo.com*
Metasearch Engines	**URL**
Dogpile	*www.dogpile.com*
Google	*www.google.com*
MetaCrawler	*metacrawler.com*
Perfect Market	*www.perfectmarket.com*

findings spurred search engine companies to increase the size of their databases, and within months many search engines claimed to have doubled or tripled their size (Sherman, 2000). The popularity of search engines tends to wax and wane over time. A useful site to check for a listing of current search engines, reviews and ratings, and tips on searching is *www.searchenginewatch.com.*

In addition to search engines, there are metasearch engines. What is the difference? A metasearch engine conducts a search of several databases from other search tools, and thus it covers more of the Web. There are two ways in which a metasearch engine approaches a search: sequentially or simultaneously. Those that perform simultaneous database searches eliminate duplicate hits (Sparks & Rizzolo, 1998).

There are also differences in the way search engines decide which Web pages or documents to include in the search findings and in which order. For example, Google looks at connections between Web sites, and the sites with the most links to them are elevated to the top of the search list (Taylor, 2000). AltaVista ranks sites based on how many times your search term is mentioned on the Web page, and the pages with the most citations of the term are placed at the top of the search list (Kiley, 1999). Because each search engine uses different databases and different techniques for searching them, it may be a good idea to use more than one tool if you want to do an exhaustive search.

SUBJECT DIRECTORIES

A variety of Internet subject directories are also available to help you search. Many search tools have a list of subject directories on their home page. If you want information about a health-related topic, for instance, you can access a Health directory and start your search at that point. Kiley (1999) makes the analogy that a subject directory is to a search engine as a book's table of contents is to a book's index. That is, you consult a table of contents (subject directory) when you want an overview of the book's contents. You consult a book index (search engine in this case) when you want to look for a specific term. Both approaches are useful for different searches.

BASIC SEARCH TECHNIQUES

If you are looking for a particular Web site, you can try to guess the URL for the site using what you know about domain names. For example, .com refers to commercial sites. Educational sites are the .edu domain, and government sites are .gov. Nonprofit agencies are .org (although some commercial sites are also .org), and foreign country sites usually end in that country's two letter code (example, .ca for Canada and .uk for United Kingdom). So, if you want to find a Web page for melanoma, you might try *www.melanoma.com* just by guessing, and lo and behold, a melanoma page pops up!

If you are looking up a key word and hope to find a number of sites that contain it, you would probably use a search engine. There are a few strategies that will help you streamline your search and get the best sites on the top of the search list. While some search techniques are unique to certain search tools, there are also some that are universal.

Most engines use Boolean logic for their searches. The term *Boolean* comes from the name of a British mathematician, George Boole, who wrote about logical relationships among search terms.

The three Boolean operators are AND, OR, and NOT. Let's use an example. If you want to find information about congestive heart failure, you could just type the three keywords—Congestive Heart Failure—with spaces between them into a search screen. In this case, the search engine will default to either AND or OR between the words, depending on the engine. (The Help file on the search engine will inform you as to which operator it uses by default and how to change it if you wish.) The operator AND narrows a search by retrieving only records that contain all three keywords. The operator OR expands the search by retrieving records that contain all or at least one of the keywords. If you want to spread your net as wide as possible, OR is the way to go. If you are interested only in records that contain the exact phrase Congestive Heart Failure, use the AND operator. The third Boolean operator is NOT. This also helps to limit your search. If you want to find documents about Ulcerative Colitis, you could try typing "Ulcerative Colitis NOT Crohns", to eliminate sites that speak to both inflammatory bowel conditions. However, be aware that by eliminating sites with Crohns in the title, you may be eliminating some valuable information about Ulcerative Colitis as well.

There are a few other search symbols that can help to control a search. First, if you place quotation marks around "Ulcerative Colitis," the search engine searches for these words as a phrase in the given word order. Second, some search engines use implied Boolean operators in place of AND, OR, and NOT. The implied operators are plus (+) and minus (−) signs used in place of AND and NOT. Usually you have to leave a space between the first word and the implied operator; for example, "Ulcerative Colitis" −Crohns. Third, some engines permit the use of wildcards. These are symbols such as * or # that are placed at the end of a truncated word in order to allow the search engine to complete the word in a variety of ways. For instance, you may type in the stem inflam* in order to retrieve references to terms like *inflammation, inflammatory,* and *inflamed.* One last tip for basic searching—many search engines are not case specific, meaning that it does not matter if you capitalize words or not. Each search engine has a Help screen or an icon for search directions that will tell you the basic search rules.

ADVANCED SEARCH TECHNIQUES

To make a search very efficient, you may choose to do an *advanced search.* Advanced search options vary somewhat with different search tools, but they offer some useful devices. For example, you may be able to limit your search to certain domain names such as .edu or .gov. You might use that technique when searching for a continuing education course. If you only want information on courses offered by educational institutions, use of .edu would eliminate all the .com or commercial continuing education sites. In an advanced search, you may also be able to limit your search to certain years, or languages, or type of site such as text or multimedia.

One last hint. Whatever means you use to find useful sites, you will eventually find some that you want to revisit frequently. You should bookmark these sites. All you have to do is click the word Bookmark on the status bar in Netscape Navigator, or Favorites in Explorer and AOL, while you are on your desired Internet site and it will save that site in memory. The next time you log on and want to retrieve that site, click Bookmark or Favorites and then click on your site name. This process saves you having to look up the URL if you don't remember it.

REFERENCES

Kiley, R. (1999). *Medical Information on the Internet*, 2d ed. Edinburgh: Churchill Livingstone.

Lawrence, S. & Giles, C. L. (1998). Searching the World Wide Web. *Science, 280*, 96, 99–100.

Sherman, C. (2000). The future revisited: What's new with Web search. *Online, 24*(3), 27–34. Retrieved June 6, 2001, from the World Wide Web: *www.onlineinc.com/onlinemag*

Sparks, S. M. & Rizzolo, M. A. (1998). World Wide Web search tools. *Image: Journal of Nursing Scholarship, 30*(2), 167–71.

Taylor, C. (2000). In search of Google. *Time, 156*(8), 66–67.

4

Being Cautious

Of the billions of Web sites, many are high quality, many are average, and many are poor. The reason for this is that there is no monitoring or quality control system for the Internet. Therefore, you must be careful in using and depending on the information at various Web sites, because the information may be very accurate and complete, but it may also be outdated, incomplete, or incorrect. So, let the user beware, and have some criteria in mind for sorting out the good from the poor. The criteria in Table 4–1 can be used to gauge the value of Web sites. Whatever information you are searching for, you can apply these criteria and have some assurance that if the site meets the standards, there is some reliability to the information.

Table 4–1	Criteria for Evaluating the Quality of WWW Sites
Purpose	1. The potential audience should be stated or obvious (i.e., for adults, children, laypeople, or professionals).
	2. The purpose or mission of the site should be stated or implied (i.e., to sell a product, provide information, etc.).
Currency	1. The site should contain up-to-date information.
	2. The pages should be updated frequently and the date of revision should be noted at the end of the pages. You can also check for the date of the most recent changes by clicking the browser's View window.

(continued)

Table 4-1	Criteria for Evaluating the Quality of WWW Sites (continued)
Credibility	1. The author's credentials should be listed and should be appropriate to the content. 2. The information for contacting the author should be listed. 3. The author's organizational affiliation should be listed, if any. 4. Anonymous sites should be handled with caution. 5. Sites sponsored by sales companies should be evaluated for their objectivity and possible conflicts of interest.
Content accuracy	1. The facts should be verifiable as being accurate and true. 2. Links to other sites should confirm the accuracy of the first. 3. The content should be logical and scientific. 4. References should be included in the site.
Design	1. Pages should be simple, not too cluttered with graphics or boxes. 2. An internal search engine and site map should be included for comprehensive sites. 3. It should be easy to move around the site without getting lost. 4. Links to other sites should be useful and you should be able to return from the linked site.

CRITERIA FOR EVALUATING WWW SITES

When these criteria are applied, you can avoid some of the pitfalls that exist on the WWW. These pitfalls include quackery, bias, and incorrect information (Kiley, 2000). You may be willing to use Web sites that include some of these flaws if you are just a curious seeker, but if you are looking for information to apply to patient care, the stakes are higher, and you will not want to take many risks.

Quackery sometimes exists on commercial (.com) Web sites. Companies that claim their products will remove all symptoms or cure all ills are suspect. Unfortunately, these claims are often disguised by the medical information that is also on the site. The medical information about the health condition may be accurate or at least plausible, but that doesn't mean the product's claims are. Use the criteria in Table 4–1 to evaluate the Purpose, Credibility, and Content accuracy of the information.

Bias is another pitfall. When researchers publish their findings in journals, they indicate whether anyone has financially supported the study. That helps the reader to be cautious in interpreting the findings, especially if the results are in favor of the supporting company's product. But on the Internet, companies providing financial support for a product or Web site may not be listed, or they may be difficult to find on the site. Again, using the criteria for Credibility in Table 4–1, you can look for signs of bias.

Incorrect information can occur in any medium, so the nurse must be careful in reading any articles or looking at any audiovisuals that include information that is going to be put to use in some way. The same prudence should be used in evaluating information on the Web. It is easy to be lured by a glitzy Web site, or a very official-looking site, into thinking that this must be a reliable site because it looks good. Some Web sites actually have awards listed on them. But those awards are often for appearance, not content. So look at content closely, using the Content accuracy criteria in Table 4–1.

Not all Internet information is free. If a site requires you to register, find out if there is a monetary charge. If there is, the site should make clear how much it is and exactly what you get for your money.

In addition, in order to view portions of some sites, you may need an operating system or plug-in that you do not have. You may first have to download a plug-in like Quick-Time or Real-Audio to view certain graphics or play multimedia segments. You must decide if you want to spend the time and effort to download those files.

For further information about evaluating Web sites, check:

www.virtualsalt.com/evalu8it.htm ****

This site is very comprehensive and has been around since 1997.

A site that is very helpful in checking for health quackery is:

www.quackwatch.com **

This site gives factual information that brings various types of quackery into question. It has been around since 1997 and is updated frequently by a physician.

Another service you can use that has already done some Web site evaluation for you is the Health on the Net Foundation (HON). This nonprofit organization, founded in 1995, is dedicated to guiding people to reliable health information on the Internet. From their Web site, *www.hon.ch*, you can search the WWW through MedHunt and HONselect to find trustworthy medical information for laypersons and professionals. There certainly may be reliable Web sites not yet evaluated by HON, so lack of endorsement doesn't necessarily mean these sites are not good, but for those sites that carry the HON seal of approval, you can have confidence in the information found there.

PRIVACY ISSUES

For most Americans, the right to privacy is strongly held. The issue of personal privacy is closely linked to personal security whether in face-to-face or computer environments. Privacy can be defined as a state or condition of inaccessibility. Computers have not changed our desire for privacy, but the limits of dissemination of information have virtually melted away.

The Internet has enabled people to access "tons" of information at the click of a mouse. When we want information, we love the speed, comprehensiveness, and ubiquity of the Internet and electronic data transfer. When we want to remain "inaccessible," the attributes of the Internet are onerous. No longer is physical access to a paper document the only way to share information. How does personal data become available to millions? The easy answer is, we give it away, often without realizing it. Every time we use a credit card, become a group member, or even request information over the Internet, we have left a bit of personal information.

One way that we give information away is when our computer and, by extension, we ourselves accept "cookies" from Internet sites. Cookies are bits of electronic data that pass from the Web server to your browser and serve as a marker of your visit to the Web site. Then, the site gets a message from this cookie every time you re-enter its site, or even certain other sites. In essence, your every move on the Internet is being followed and recorded somewhere. These trails are purchased in some cases and "hacked" (stolen) in other cases. This data, combined with your real identity information, is shared when you gain access to a site or place an order, and places you in the position of being public. Gathering data from public and private resources is a booming business, whether on the Internet or elsewhere.

In 1999, a Georgetown University study revealed that nine out of ten commercial Web sites asked their users to supply at least one piece of personal information, such as your name, e-mail address, or postal address before gaining access to their site (Tynan, 2000). This information is used to develop consumer profiles. They may use cookies to see what entertainment and travel preferences you researched as well as the health conditions or disease-specific sites you visited. "This information could be added to the user's profile, and employers could lower their insurance premiums by not hiring employees who could potentially have serious illnesses" (Tynan, 2000, p. 106). Further, Richard Smith (cited in Tynan, 2000) reported that numerous health sites share visitors' personal data without their consent.

How can you protect yourself? A few tweaks to your Internet browser can make you a lot less accessible, although complete privacy is impossible today. *PC World* (2000) suggests that you check your browser's level of encryption. Encryption is a technology that scrambles the information between your computer and another computer or Internet site. The greater the number of bits, the better the security. The default setting on most browsers is 40 to 56 bits. Most authorities believe that 1024 bits is best, but the more bits used in encrypting, the slower your computer will process. A very slow data exchange can be frustrating and lead a person to abandon encryption for speed. There are a number of software applications to help protect your privacy in the online environment. See *PC World* (June 2000) for reviews.

Both Netscape and Internet Explorer browsers allow you to select to be "warned" before accepting a "cookie" or any executable file. You can set this by clicking Internet Options in the Tools or File area of your browser's menu bar. Under Options, open the Security folder and look for Cookies. You may select to decline (disable) all cookies, accept all cookies, or prompt all cookies. If you choose prompt, you will realize just how many cookies are being placed on your computer. Most browsers default to accept all cookies and the owner never really thinks about it. You can often decline the cookie and still gain access to the site; however, some sites will not allow you to enter.

AOL is a favorite of computer hackers because they have the most subscribers among all ISPs. Hackers can get your name and profile from chat rooms you visit, as well as Web sites you access. The information is sold to SPAMers (unsolicited e-mail distributors) or used to send unsolicited Instant Messages asking for "password verification," thus enabling them to access your account surreptitiously.

In addition, remember that you should not put anything in an e-mail message that you would not put on a postcard. E-mail is not secure. Do not use or accept e-mail that is HTML coded. It may contain viruses, Trojan horses, or malicious Java scripts that can inhabit your computer and perform unknown annoying or even illegal activities.

There are a lot of issues related to authenticity, reliability, privacy, and security when using the WWW. But, don't let your fears keep you from participating in the many benefits that this easily accessible, vast source of information provides. You can become a much better informed nurse and your patients can obtain much needed relationships with you and "good" information, if you use critical thinking and a few controls on your browser.

REFERENCES

Kiley, R. (2000). *Medical Information on the Internet*, 2d ed. Edinburgh: Churchill Livingstone.

Tynan, D. (2000). Privacy 2000: In web we trust? *PC World, 18*(6), 112.

Selecting Courses

After graduating from a nursing program, no nurse can afford to stop learning. But if you are working and raising a family or have other responsibilities, it isn't easy to travel around to continuing education programs or college courses. If you are looking for educational opportunities and want to increase your range of choices and flexibility of scheduling, you may want to look to the Web.

TYPES OF COURSES

Some courses are offered totally online. Some have partial online components. Courses (whether for credit or CE units) run the gamut in terms of online involvement, and you have a lot of choice as to the type of course you want.

First, there are courses that are completely online. You will never meet the teacher or other students in person. You may meet them online in planned topical discussions, sometimes called threaded discussions, or in chat rooms, or you may even see pictures of them online. You can also converse individually with them by e-mail. However, it is also possible to have an online course where you independently complete the coursework and never contact another student.

Second, there are courses that are mostly online but include some visits to the campus or sponsoring institution. The visits are often at the beginning of the course, when examinations are given, and possibly a debriefing session at the end. In some cases, especially with credit courses offered by large universities, there are central locations around the country where students meet with preceptors or local coordinators periodically throughout the course.

Third, courses that are more traditional in nature may include an online component that enhances the learning experience. For instance, there may be online discussions that take place in addition to classroom discussions, or course materials are posted and can be downloaded from the Web site. There may also be Internet-based assignments that replace some in-class assignments. Obviously, this last type of course provides the least flexibility and requires the closest geographic proximity.

Whether you take a course for college credit or continuing education units (CEUs) will be determined by your goals. If you wish to earn a graduate degree you would, of course, take courses for credit within a degree program. If you wish to earn a certificate in a specialty, your courses will generally be noncredit or CEU courses, although some certificate programs do require or accept credit-bearing courses. If you are not aiming toward a graduate degree or a certificate, you probably want to take continuing education courses or programs for CEUs.

EVALUATING SUITABILITY OF COURSES AND PROGRAMS

Courses and programs are available to you through colleges and universities, private continuing education companies, professional organizations such as the American Nurses Association, and textbook publishers. Your decision about what courses to take should include deliberations about a number of variables. These include cost, quality, nature of provider, and whether the course meets your professional needs.

Online college or university courses are often more expensive than traditional courses because they require expensive technological support. Your transportation savings, however, may offset the increased cost. In contrast, many online programs offered for CEUs are quite inexpensive. The provider may actually allow you to complete the offering for free, but it you want to receive a CEU certificate, you pay a nominal fee such as $12 to $15.

Indicators, such as accreditation or reputation of the provider, resources and support offered to learners, and satisfaction levels of former course-takers, can help you judge the quality of courses and programs. If you are thinking of taking a credit-bearing course, make sure it is offered by an accredited institution. In nursing, that generally means being accredited by the Commission on Collegiate Nursing Education or the National League for Nursing. If the program is given totally by distance learning, it may not be accredited yet by a nursing organization, but should have at least regional accreditation by a group like the Southern Regional Education Board or the Middle States Association of Colleges and Secondary Schools. If you are taking a continuing education program for CEUs, make sure an approved provider or an official organization such as a state nurses' association or the American Nurses Credentialling Center is giving the CEUs. You must also know, or be able to find out, something about the reputation of the provider. If the provider is a well-known university, you will have a high level of confidence in the quality of the offering. Or, if the provider is a well-known national organization, they are most likely to stand behind the quality of their programs.

Before committing yourself to an online course or program, you should find out what resources and technological support are available to you. Are library resources available, both online and in-person? How are arrangements made for library resources? How do you access technology support? If you have difficulty accessing course materials or using the Web platform, is help readily available? How accessible will the instructor be? Is there scheduled time for e-mail or phone calls to the instructor? Lack of adequate support can make the learning experience very frustrating, so it is important to find out what is made available to you. If you take an online continuing education offering, support may not be as important. Many offerings are comprised of online journal articles with a post-test that you take for CEUs. Others may require you to read an online article and visit a variety of related Web sites or to view audiovisual software that may be housed in a library.

It may be possible to find out something about satisfaction levels of previous customers. Ask if there is a former student with whom you can communicate. It is also worth asking if there is a money back guarantee in case you are not satisfied. Guarantees are sometimes advertised by private continuing education companies, but rarely by institutions of higher education.

In addition to quality issues, there are considerations about the suitability of the course to meet your purposes. Look for information about the intended audience for the course. If you are an experienced critical care nurse, you would probably not want to take a course on ventilators, for example, that says it is intended for generalist nurse audiences. If your aim is to become more expert in your field, look carefully for indications that the course is for specialists. If you are seeking credit-bearing courses that may eventually lead to a degree, do some research to find out if this course is likely to transfer into a degree program.

ARE DISTANCE LEARNING COURSES FOR YOU?

Online learning is not for everyone. Although most people may like the fact that they can learn in the comfort of their homes at any time of day or night, that doesn't mean an online course is the right fit for every learner. Because we have different learning styles, preferred ways of interacting in the learning situation, and varying needs for structure in learning, we may all have slightly different reactions to distance learning. The characteristics thought to be necessary for a successful distance learning student can be seen in Table 5–1. In general, you need to be self-disciplined, be able to structure your own learning to a great extent, and be comfortable without face-to-face contact with a teacher and other students. You will probably not be very successful in an online course if you are a serious procrastinator. The following Web sites can also be consulted for personal qualities needed to enhance success in online courses:

illinois.online.uillinois.edu/model/studentprofile.htm
www.petersons.com/dlearn/study.html

Table 5–1	Characteristics That Increase Likelihood of Success in Distance Learning Courses

1. *Self-discipline:* No one is going to tell you that you have to go online and do the coursework. You must set aside time for the work.

2. *Computer literacy:* You must have the appropriate proficiency needed to negotiate the course platform, and the necessary computer hardware.

3. *Writing skill:* In most courses, you have not only traditional writing assignments, but also written discussions, and possibly group work online.

4. *Communication skill:* The ability to think ahead and marshal one's thoughts before responding is important, and will enhance the quality of threaded discussions.

5. *Independence:* You won't be going to class but learning, for the most part, on your own. Can you survive without face-to-face interactions and the camaraderie of a classroom?

6. *Self-confidence in learning:* You're on your own more than you are in a traditional classroom. If you are having difficulty in any part of the course, you have to speak up, because the teacher cannot read your body language.

LOCATING ONLINE COURSES AND PROGRAMS

You could conduct an Internet search to find appropriate courses or programs (see Chapter 3 for how to conduct the search). If you know you would like to take a college or university sponsored course, you can find the URL for the institution and then click on their Continuing Education division. You can also type in the URL for a nursing organization with which you are familiar and see if they offer online programs. Chapter 6 contains a listing of popular continuing education Web sites.

6

World Wide Web Sites and Their Ratings†

ALLERGY

The Allergy Center

www.onlineallergycenter.com ****
Information designed for allergy sufferers. Includes information about allergies in general, airborne allergies, hormone allergies, asthma, and food allergies. Also covers topics like ear infections, sinusitis, nasal irrigation, and air cleaners.

Allergy Internet Resources

www.Immune.Com/allergy/allabc.html ***
A collection of links on allergy topics such as asthma, food allergies, kid's allergies, latex allergy, hay fever and seasonal allergies, skin allergies, stings, and anaphylaxis. Within those categories are subtopics like finding asthma triggers, teaching your patients about asthma, and an asthma tutorial. Includes a discussion group.

Asthma & Allergy Case Studies

www.hopkins-allergy.org/case_studies ***
Site developed by Johns Hopkins School of Medicine. Case studies are searchable by symptoms, age group, or key words. Each case study includes chief complaints, history and physical findings, lab

† Note: Ratings range from a low of * to a high of *****

studies and recommendation for treatment. Links to other sites are available for prescribing information.

ALTERNATIVE AND COMPLEMENTARY MEDICINE

The Alternative Medicine HomePage

www.pitt.edu/~cbw/altm.html ****
A University of Pittsburgh page designed to give information on alternative therapies like biofeedback, herbal medicine, diet, homeopathy, New Age healing, chiropractic, acupuncture, naturopathy, magnets, massage, and music and prayer therapy. Includes information on fraud and quackery. Includes links to diseases that may be helped with alternative medicine.

Alternative/Complementary Medicine

www.wellweb.com/alternativecomplementary_medicine.htm ****
A general resource site of alternative/complementary medicine topics such as cancer prevention and treatment, herbs and supplements, and other nutritional approaches. Includes general information on choosing health insurance plans and also includes information on quackery.

National Center for Complementary and Alternative Medicine

nccam.nih.gov *****
Contains fact sheets on therapies plus research being conducted at NIH (clinical trials and clinical studies). Also focuses on Consensus Reports, and Complementary and Alternative Medicine databases.

Rosenthal Center

cpmcnet.columbia.edu/dept/rosenthal/About_us.html ***
A center at Columbia University's medical school. Their primary mission is research in complementary/alternative medicine. Under "Information Resources" you can find basic information, FAQs, and clinical trials. Includes links to related sites.

ANATOMY AND PHYSIOLOGY

Acid-Base Tutorial

www.tmc.tulane.edu/departments/anesthesiology/acid/default. html ***

This site provides a detailed explanation and rationale of Acid-Base Balance. The Department of Anesthesiology of Tulane University School of Medicine has developed it. It is not for the non-scientific mind. However, the author does have a sense of humor, for example, picture of a flame to describe the waste products of fire as analogous to the waste products of metabolism, that is, CO_2.

Anatomy/Physiology

biology.about.com/science/biology/mbody.htm *****

Click Anatomy and Physiology for detailed information on organs and body systems. Excellent review of body systems. Dissection slides available. Virtual dissection is available. Also includes information on cell anatomy and cell biology. Includes links to related sites.

Brain Links

snow.utoronto.ca/Learn2/resources/brain.html *****

An extensive set of links to sites to learn about the brain. Includes imaging of the brain, information on disorders and diseases, research, IQ tests, and a brain puzzle, plus many other resources. Includes a link to the Whole Brain Atlas project at Harvard. You can see what the brain looks like in dementia, stroke, and so on.

David, Online Atlas of Human Anatomy

www.cid.ch/DAVID/Mainmenu.html ****

Site developed by J. C. Oberson of the Diagnostic Imaging Center of Lausanne, Switzerland. Click any area of the body diagrams for more information about that part and continue clicking on diagram labels or within the image itself for finer details and labeling. You can also click Index Classification or Thematic Classification to shortcut to the area of the anatomy for which you want information.

Department of Dermatology—University of Iowa

tray.dermatology.uiowa.edu/DermImag.htm ****
Extensive database of dozens of skin disease photographs, including rare conditions. Photographs are very clear.

Dermatology Image Bank

www-medlib.med.utah.edu/kw/derm ***
From the University of Utah Medical Library. Tutorials on topics like anatomy and physiology of the skin, melanoma, keratoses, squamous carcinoma, infections, acne vulgaris, dermatitis, hair, and nails. For each topic, includes overview and detail photographs, definition, incidence, etiology, symptoms and signs, treatment, and cost of treatment. Also includes a 100-item self-quiz.

Digestive System

arbl.cvmbs.colostate.edu/hbooks/pathphys/digestion ***
Although this is entitled "pathophysiology," it is actually a good tutorial and review on physiology of the digestive system with good diagrams and motion models. Focuses on "A Voyage Through the Digestive Track." Each part of the anatomy is explained in detail and related topics are found at the end of each section. For example, under the Liver topic, there is information about regeneration of the liver and development of gallstones.

Digital Anatomist Project

www9.biostr.washington.edu/ ****
Site of the University of Washington. Anatomy of the heart, lungs, brain, and knee with models, dissections, and x-rays. 3-D and 2-D views are shown from MRI scans, cadaver dissections, and computer reconstructions.

Human Reproduction

www-medlib.med.utah.edu/kw/human_reprod ****
From the University of Utah Medical Library. Course materials on Human Reproduction. Includes lectures on topics like Prolactin Physiology, Pubertal and Midlife Changes, Ovarian Lifecycle, Infertility, Gyn Disorders, Physiology of Normal Labor and Delivery, and Clinical Genetics. Also has clinical case studies and slides and movies.

Hypermuscle: Muscles in Action

www.med.umich.edu:80/lrc/Hypermuscle/Hyper.html ****
Great program for learning range of motion and types of muscle action. Needs Quick Time to see video action, but even without it, positions are demonstrated with photographs and described in the narrative.

Inner Learning Online: Human Anatomy Online

www.innerbody.com/default.htm *****
Illustrations of anatomic structures with animation. Click any part of an anatomical structure and receive information about it on the side of the screen. Good for beginners and young learners because of the interactive nature, but a useful and interesting review for anyone.

Integrated Medical Curriculum

www.imc.gsm.com/siteinfo/whatis.htm ****
Registration required, but free. Contains images of cadaver dissection that can be used for simulated laboratories, anatomy as seen on x-rays (CT, MRI and plain film), and information on basic physiology and immunology. Also includes a quiz feature.

Lumen Dissector

www.meddean.luc.edu/lumen/meded/grossanatomy/dissector/index.html *****
From Loyola University Medical College. Course materials for Structure of the Human Body. Wonderful tutorials on anatomy, broken down by major areas of the body such as back, upper extremity, head and neck, thorax, abdomen, and so on. In each body area, there are objectives, concepts, tutorials, cross-sections by CT and MRIs, and practice examinations.

Master Muscle List

www.meddean.luc.edu/lumen/MedEd/GrossAnatomy/dissector/mml/index.htm ****
An excellent view and explanation of all body muscles. Access muscles by anatomic region or alphabetically. Includes information on origin, insertion, nerve supply, and action. Selecting an individual muscle will display an illustration of the muscle along with related functional information.

Radiographic Anatomy of the Skeleton

www.scar.rad.washington.edu/Rad/Anatomy.html ***
University of Washington site. Plain x-ray images of various parts
of the skeletal system (two or three views of each bone or joint).
Click the x-ray to get a labeled version.

Science Education Site: Adam Software

www.adam.com/home.htm ***
A site that will entice you. It is a repository for the programs titled
Adam. These are available in software stores or can be purchased
online. This site offers 6-month subscriptions of online access to
some of the programs. A more cost effective way to supplement
your Physiology course. The Anatomy CD is simplistic from a
nurse's point of view, but the visuals may be helpful in developing
teaching materials for patients.

The X-ray Files

www.radiology.co.uk/xrayfile/xray/info/intro.htm ****
British site. X-rays can be viewed relative to patient cases. The patient history and an x-ray image are presented and questions are
posed about it. Answers are also given. The tutorials (on conditions like renal transplants, lobar collapse of the lung, and head
trauma) are excellent.

CARE PLANS

Care Plan Corner

rncentral.com ***
Contains a very nice standard care plan format that can be adapted
for individual use online and can be printed. Just click the options
that are provided in the diagnosis and intervention boxes. Also contains problem statements and symptoms, a chat room, and a library.

Care Plan Resource Center

www.careplans.com ***
A site built by nurses. The "Library" contains an alphabetical list
of problem statements and useful reference sources such as MDS.
Also includes a real-time chat room and discussion forums to en-
courage sharing of ideas and resources on care planning.

Links to Care Plans and Case Studies

www.iun.edu/Libemb/nursing/careplan.htm **

Site developed by a librarian at Indiana University. Some useful links for care plans, but some links may be outdated (some links are from other colleges and universities). Includes some sample care plan sites, and links to care plan software.

Nursing Care Plans/Nursing Process/Nursing Diagnoses

www.nursing.about.com/health/msubplans.htm *****

Contains a list of links to sites on these topics. This site is part of the About.com series (previously called The Mining Company). Contains many excellent resources, including basic information on writing care plans, NANDA nursing diagnoses, sample care plans, and reference sources.

COMMUNITY HEALTH NURSING

American Academy of Ambulatory Care Nursing

aaacn.inurse.com:80 ***

Site of this organization. Has information on the organization, its mission, goals, and benefits. There is a list of special interest groups. Contains clinical practice standards for telephone nursing, ambulatory care nursing, and administration. Also includes information on certification and an examination preparation guide.

American Public Health Association

www.apha.org ****

Information on the association, news, and legislative issues. Also includes lists of state public health associations, information on the World Federation of Public Health Associations, and public health links. Some links are not functioning. Continuing education information provided.

CDC Prevention Guidelines Database

aepo-xdv-www.epo.cdc.gov/wonder/prevguid/prevguid.shtml ***

Sponsored by the Centers for Disease Control. Site enables you to search the CDC Prevention Guidelines and access a topic list and title list alphabetically or by date. Includes over 400 documents on prevention of diseases, disabilities, and injuries. Also includes a directory of state public health directors.

Department of Health and Human Services Health Statistics

ncvhs.hhs.gov ****

The National Committee on Vital and Health Statistics of the U.S. Department of Health and Human Services has compiled this excellent site of information related to Federal support of health initiatives. Includes health data and statistics.

Florida Tobacco Control Clearinghouse

www.ftcc.fsu.edu ****

Sponsored by the Florida Department of Health. Includes links to publications, videos, and CDs that discourage smoking. Also includes news, events, legislation, a speaker's bureau, and a chat room. Funding opportunities are also listed.

Healthy People

www.health.gov/healthypeople *****

Sponsored by the U.S. Department of Health and Human Services. Overview of Healthy People 2010 with history, goals, and implementation plans. The leading health indicators are listed. Information on how to order the 2010 publications is given.

Home Healthcare Nurses Association

www.nahc.org/HHNA **

Site of the organization, with information on membership, events, news, and products. Relevant to those in home health clinical practice, education, administration, or research.

Morbidity and Mortality Weekly Report

www.cdc.gov/mmwr ****

This is a publication of the Centers for Disease Control. The sites contains data on morbidity and mortality tables reported by the 50 states. Fact sheets are also available on many public health related diseases, accidents, and conditions. International bulletins and information on publications are also included.

Occupational Safety and Health Administration

www.osha.gov ****
Information about OSHA's mission and the OSHA Act of 1970. Also includes programs and services, and OSHA facts and statistics. A Library and News Room is included. A resource for workers page includes an electronic filing system for complaints.

CONSUMER HEALTH INFORMATION

The Breast Self-Exam

www.lhj.com/health/cancer/knowbrst.htm ****
Part of the Ladies Home Journal page. Includes illustrations of how to perform self-breast exam. Includes FAQs about SBE and a self-exam video. Also information about "lumps and bumps" and risk factors. Link to breast cancer site.

CBS Health Watch

cbshealthwatch.medscape.com/medscape/p/gcommunity/ghome21.asp *****
A portal through Medscape to a wide range of consumer health information. There are 46 Health Channels on topics like asthma, heart health, mental health, reproductive health, and weight management. Health topics are also listed A–Z. There is a drug directory, a medical dictionary, a weight loss center, a marketplace for health and beauty and sports and fitness. Health news is included and discussion boards. Features an Ask an Expert opportunity.

Health A to Z.com

www.healthatoz.com ****
All types of information for consumers. Information on health for men and women and all age groups. Forums with information on various diseases and conditions. Information on alternative medicine, fitness, and healthful lifestyles. Includes some tools to measure body mass index, target heart rate, due date, and kid's growth.

Healthfinder

www.healthfinder.gov *****
Produced by the U.S. Office of Disease Prevention and Health Promotion, it is a portal to many sources of information for con-

sumers on diseases and illnesses. Searches can be narrowed by age group or population. Includes "hot topics" in the news and information on health promotion and self-care. Links to support groups and listservs are provided. Spanish language is available.

Health Seek

www.healthseek.com ****
A portal to a variety of sites for consumers and professionals. Includes links to a directory of physician groups, professional organizations, nutrition sites, pharmaceuticals, and medical databases. Also includes discussion groups for nurses and physicians.

Healthtouch

www.healthtouch.com/level1/hi_toc.htm ****
Extensive alphabetical list of diseases and conditions. Information is provided by professional organizations in the form of pamphlets you can download and distribute. Bibliographic sources are given for each pamphlet (there may be several for some diseases).

InteliHealth

www.intelihealth.com/IH *****
Sponsored by Harvard Medical School, this is a valuable source of information on common disease conditions (listed alphabetically) for consumers. Healthy Living information is provided. Cool Tools are a group of interactive learning tools on a variety of health topics. Also provides access to the U.S. Pharmacopeia for drug information for consumers. You can search the drug database by trade or generic name or go through an alphabetical list of drugs.

Patient Resources on the Internet

www.gahec.org/library/pated.htm **
One of many compilations of patient education and consumer health resources on the Internet. This one is provided and compiled by Greensboro Area Health Education Centers in North Carolina.

Yahoo Health

dir.yahoo.com/health/index.html ****
A directory of health-related categories listed alphabetically. Topics range from alternative medicine, to diseases and conditions, to

first aid, to men's health and weight issues. Clicking a topic leads to further breakdown in categories and ultimately to Web sites.

CONTINUING EDUCATION

American Nurses Credentialing Center (ANCC)

www.nursingworld.org/ancc/index.htm *****
This is the branch of the American Nurses Association that accredits continuing education providers. Click on information about certification exams. Many continuing education offerings are available. Earn online CEUs instantly when CE offerings are completed.

Buchanan & Associates Continuing Education Credits for RNs

www.nursingce.com **
Approved provider of continuing education by ANCC, California and Florida boards of nursing. Offers articles in many nursing specialties. The process is to fill out the order form for the articles you want ($12 per article). Read the article, complete the multiple-choice test, and mail it in. Articles usually carry 1 to 2 CEUs per article. You will receive the CEU certificate by mail.

CE-web

www.ce-web.com ***
Approved provider of continuing education by ANCC and ACCME. Offers articles and tests on 18 topics, each about 1 to 2 contact hours. Tests cost under $15 (discount on bulk orders).

Concept Media

www.conceptmedia.com/ce.htm ***
Approved provider of continuing education by the California Board of Registered Nursing. Procedure is to request a test online or by phone for the subjects offered on the list. The list contains Concept Media video programs and CD-ROM programs. You must view the software in an institutional setting, then complete the test and mail it in with $5 for each hour of CE. Most of the software contains 1.5 to 2 hours of CE.

Drug Store News

www.drugstorenews.com ***
Approved provider of continuing education by the American Council on Pharmaceutical Education. Provides clinical pharmacology information on a variety of conditions. Process is to click on the lesson you want, read the article, take the test, and submit it online or by mail with $6.95 per lesson.

MEDCEU

medceu.com ****
Approved provider of continuing education by ANCC. Offers over 100 articles online. Click on a course you want, read the material, and take the post-test. You only pay if you pass the test and want CEUs. Then the fee is $9.95 per credit. Receive CEU certificate online. This site also offers a Personal Professional Planner. Register free and the planner will tell you your state's requirements, and will keep track of your CEUs and keep a copy of your certificates.

Medcom, Inc.

www.medcominc.com/cgi-bin/mc/index ****
Approved provider of continuing education by ANCC. Provides CE courses online in 20 clinical areas. Most courses are 1 to 2 hours and cost $5 per contact hour. Courses are rated by previous users and average ratings are provided. Courses include printed material, as well as linking you to imbedded sites for diagrams, x-rays, and so on. (One problem is that you cannot always return from these sites.) Also provides information on conferences.

NPACE

www.npace.org/about.htm **
Continuing education for Nurse Practitioners across multidisciplinary specialties. Traditionally, CE was offered through conferences. Just began online continuing education with a program on vulvar dermatology.

Nursing Center.com

www.nursingcenter.com *****
Contains 203 online articles with online tests. Cost is $8 for 1 hour of continuing education. Also offers interactive CE, where all an-

swers are correct and reflect your level of expertise, from novice to expert. Offers Nursing Rounds based on actual case histories, or Knowledge Quest where you read a full text journal article and then seek further knowledge by visiting specified Web sites. Receive instant test results and a CE certificate.

Nursing Online Continuing Education (CEUs) on: The Nurse Friendly

www.nursefriendly.com/nursing/linksections/continuing education.htm ***
A list of links to online nursing education providers such as American Nurses Credentialling Center, AORN, Buchanan & Associates, Center for Health Education, Mayo Continuing Nursing Education, Medcom, Professional Education Center, Free Nursing CEUs, and so on. Some links are not active.

RnCeus.com

www.rnceus.com/index.html ****
Approved provider of continuing education by ANCC. Offers 20 interactive online courses that include sound and motion. Most courses are 3 to 4 hours and cost about $4 per hour. Tests and CEU certificates are handled online.

RNWeb

www.RNWeb.com ***
Site of *RN* journal's continuing education offerings. Approved provider of continuing education by ANCC. Many topics are offered. Select an article, take the test, and pay $15. Each article is 2 contact hours. CEU certificates are available online.

CRITICAL CARE NURSING

ACLS

www.randylarson.com/acls ***
Good site for Advanced Cardiac Life Support information and practice tests, including a brief ACLS multiple-choice exam. Includes practice with rhythms, information on drugs, and a test megacode. A message board for comments and questions is available.

ACLS Algorithms

www.cardiac.org/aclsalgr.html **

A complete copy of ACLS algorithms as published in *Volume I ACLS Certification Preparation*, 3d ed., by Grauer and Cavallaro, 1993.

American Association of Critical Care Nurses

www.aacn.org *****

Contains information on AACN services, publications, and certification. There are also threaded discussions on a variety of critical care clinical topics that look very helpful. You can get answers to your pressing clinical questions.

Critical Care Nursing

www.wwnurse.com/nursing/criticalcare.shtml **

List of links to critical care organizations and critical care information Web pages and an emergency medicine site. Also links to nursing books and jobs.

Critical Care References

www.a-ten.com/alz/ccrt.htm **

A potentially useful list of review books for critical care certification. Click the book links for purchase information.

Donor Services

korrnet.org/donors ***

Contains good factual information on organ donation, with FAQs, statistics, and religious positions on organ transplantation. You can request a donor card on this site. Also includes links to related sites.

Emergency Nursing World!

ENW.org:80 ***

Site of the Emergency Nursing World organization. Includes information about the organization, plus links to research and clinical articles such as "End Tidal CO_2 Monitoring in CPR," "The Ten Commandments on Airway Maintenance," and "Principles for Sedated Position." Also has links to related sites.

ICUSTAT

icustat.com ***
A site committed to providing health care providers with information related to critical care. Good links to top health care sites. Information about continuing education is included, as well as a chat room for professionals. The Learn CPR button contains a good review of basic CPR.

MD Choice

mdchoice.com/main.asp *****
A portal to all kinds of medical and nursing information for professionals and consumers. Enter a topic and select the type of information you want to view. Includes "photo rounds," which are cases with photographs. Also includes the "Cyber-Patient Simulator" with excellent interactive critical care simulations.

Trauma Moulage

www.trauma.org/resus/moulage/moulage.html ****
Developed by Trauma Org, an organization with a mission to disseminate information about trauma prevention and treatment. These moulage pages are practice scenarios where patients are presented to be assessed and managed. The moulages include a cervical spine injury, general trauma, and pediatric trauma.

Trauma Nursing

traumaburn.com/Education.htm ***
Contains some PowerPoint slide series on topics like spinal cord injury, hypothermia in the trauma patient, acute pancreatitis, PAC removal, and cardiac complications. Also includes meeting announcements and links to a few other trauma sites.

United Network for Organ Sharing

www.unos.org/main_default.htm ****
Site of the national network for organ sharing, the world's most technologically advanced transplant system. Gives opportunity to ask for data you need. The waiting list for organs is displayed and updated weekly. News and conference information is included.

CRITICAL THINKING

California Academic Press

www.calpress.com *****
Includes descriptions of their critical thinking assessment instruments, how to score them, and order forms. Also describes their consulting services, articles about critical thinking, and related Web sites.

Critical Thinking Community

www.criticalthinking.org ***
This site is sponsored by several organizations involved in critical thinking in education. Two tracks are available, one for college and university education, the other for primary and secondary education. Provides information on events such as seminars and conferences, and resources such as curriculum guidelines and lesson plans. Also contains a library of published and unpublished writings, and a bookstore.

Critical Thinking in Nursing Education

www.cariboo.bc.ca/psd/nursing/faculty/heaslip/ct.htm **
A list of links to other Web sites on critical thinking such as Critical Thinking Centers. Also contains a page of descriptions with references on what critical thinking is in nursing education.

CULTURE

The Center for Cross Cultural Health

www.crosshealth.com/ ****
This site was created by CCHCP (Cross Cultural Health Care Program) of Seattle (and the world) according to the home page. It contains wonderful cultural resources to aid in achieving health care without barriers. The awareness for the project and Web site came from increasing numbers of immigrants finding their way to the health care system. The site is designed to help professionals. Includes curriculum outlines, multicultural training, and medical translating certification programs.

DATABASES

CDC Wonder

wonder.cdc.gov/ *****
CDC Wonder provides access to health information data sets that can be downloaded. Good for nurses interested in public health issues and for students to use in examining relationships between health and demographic data.

Centerwatch

www.centerwatch.com/ *****
A very intuitive site for identifying clinical trials being conducted in industry as well as government-sponsored trials. Provides criteria in appealing format for inclusion and contact telephone numbers and addresses. Easier than the *clinicaltrials.gov* site, but information seems similar.

Clinical Trials.gov

clinicaltrials.gov/ *****
This is a database of the U.S. National Institutes of Health. The site, indexed through the National Library of Medicine, provides patients, family members, health care professionals, and members of the public easy access to information on clinical trials for a wide range of diseases and conditions.

CRISP

crisp.cit.nih.gov/ ****
CRISP (Computer Retrieval of Information on Scientific Projects) is a searchable biomedical database system containing information on research projects and programs supported by the Department of Health and Human Services. Searches return grant number, PI name and title, project title, an abstract, institution, and dates. CRISP is updated weekly.

CINAHL Information Systems

www.cinahl.com/ ****
The Cumulative Index of Nursing and Allied Health Literature (CINAHL) is available online directly to your home computer for

a fee. This database is essential to nurses who do not have easy access at their agencies or local hospital. It is definitely easier than going to the library. There is a membership fee but worth it if you need to do research for a course.

Medscape

www.medscape.com *****
Medscape was first to provide access to Medline before the National Institutes of Health provided this service. It is still available but not as obviously as other services. The interface, however, is very pleasing and intuitive. Recommended to new users of the Medline database.

PubMed

www.ncbi.nlm.nih.gov/ *****
PubMed is a service of the United States National Library of Medicine that provides an interface to the public to the Medline database. Medline indexes over 7,000 journals in several languages to provide the most comprehensive collection of biomedical, nursing, and life science literature. A new tutorial is very helpful to a new user.

DEATH AND DYING

Death and Dying

dying.miningco.com/health/dying *****
From the former Mining Company.com, now called About.com. A lot of useful information about grief, bereavement, and comforting. Also includes articles and information on near-death experiences, advanced directives, dying at home, signs of dying, euthanasia, and funerals.

Growth House, Inc.

www.growthhouse.org *****
A portal to many resources to help people understand and deal with life-threatening illness, and death and dying. Includes information on resources for caring for the dying, guides to major illnesses, sites on grief and bereavement, and information on hospice and palliative care. There is an online bookstore and a free monthly e-mail newsletter.

Hospice Net: Bereavement

hospicenet.org/html/bereavement.html ****
Includes articles on topics like, "A Guide to Grief," "Keeping Watch," "Children and Grief," "Helping Teenagers Cope with Grief," and "Healing After a Loss." Includes general information about hospice services and related bereavement links.

EVIDENCE-BASED PRACTICE

Agency for Healthcare Research and Quality

www.ahrq.gov ****
Formerly known as the Agency for Health Care Policy and Research, this is the official government agency for providing evidence-based information on health care outcomes. Includes evidence reports, data and surveys, research findings, and funding opportunities. Quality assessment mechanisms are described. The Five Steps to Safer Health Care is impressive. The advice given is intended to make the U.S. health care system safer for patients and the public.

Best Practice Network

ww1.best4health.org/startbp.cfm ***
A place to read about and share best practices in health care and benchmarking. The site is a little difficult to navigate, but there is a lot of good information. Click Resource Center to learn about best practices and how to benchmark. To submit an abstract of best practices, click Best Practices. To share programs that work, click on that title; to share clinical guidelines, click Tools of the Trade. Also a discussion group on current topics.

Evidence-Based Health Care Resources

www.urmc.rochester.edu/Miner/Links/ebmlinks.html ****
From the University of Rochester Medical Center, a good list of links to related resources including organizations focused on evidence-based practice. Includes tutorials on evidence-based practice as well as tools, practice guidelines, and search filters.

Evidence-Based Medicine ToolKit

www.med.ualberta.ca/ebm/toc.htm ***
A useful tutorial on processes used to find and evaluate information on evidence-based practice. Includes information on searching
databases for clinical trials, and worksheets to evaluate research
and protocols.

Healthcare Advocacy

www.florenceproject.org/ ***
The Florence Project, Inc., is a nationwide nonprofit organization
that grew out of a need identified on a nursing listserv. It is com-
posed of nurses and citizens dedicated to advocating for safe,
quality health care. Their mission is to advocate and inspire nurses
to make a difference in the health care system both for patients,
and for the profession of nursing by effecting legislative and institutional policy changes. The site provides links to many articles
and legislative initiatives. There are local Web pages as well as this
national Web site. This is related to evidence-based practice because of its emphasis on quality care.

The Joanna Briggs Institute for Evidence-Based Nursing and Midwifery

joannabriggs.edu.au/welcome.html *****
Australian site that includes "best practice" information sheets on
clinical practice areas such as patient falls, tracheal suctioning,
preoperative teaching, group therapy, vital signs, and constipation.
Includes a notice board and membership information.

National Guideline Clearinghouse

www.guideline.gov/index.asp *****
The Clearinghouse is operated by the U.S. Department of Health
and Human Services, and the Agency for Healthcare Research and
Quality in partnership with the American Medical Association and
the American Association of Health Plans. It is a search site, by
topic or disease, which reveals clinical practice guidelines that are
evidence-based and available in full text. This is a fabulous site for
anyone interested in articles about your own or a patient's illness
that are research supported.

Nursing Sites on the World Wide Web: Evidence-Based Nursing

ublib.buffalo.edu/libraries/units/hsl/internet/ebn.html ****

From the University of Buffalo Library, a set of very useful links on the topic of evidence-based nursing. Includes sites for related organizations, literature appraisals, evidence-based filters for CINAHL, data sources, and search strategies to identify meta-analyses.

Pediatric Evidence-Based Medicine

depts.washington.edu/pedebm ***

Summary of evidence-based clinical topics in areas like adolescent medicine, allergy and immunology, behavior and development, genetics, infectious disease, neonatology, neurology, orthopedics, psychiatry, pulmonary medicine, rehabilitation, and surgery. Includes links to related sites.

GASTROINTESTINAL NURSING

Clinical Trials: Gastrointestinal Diseases and Disorders

www.centerwatch.com/patient/studies/cat71.html ***

A clinical trials listing service. Current clinical trials for gastrointestinal diseases and disorders are listed with links. Also includes information on clinical research in general. Includes links to other sites for information on GI problems for both professionals and patients.

Gastrointestinal Endoscopy

www.asge.org/p_body.jsp ***

A site for health professionals who work with patients undergoing endoscopy. Includes "find an endoscopist," plus patient information and a database of clinical updates and patient care guidelines.

International Foundation for Functional Gastrointestinal Disorders

www.iffgd.org ***

Site sponsored by five pharmaceutical companies. Information on functional problems like irritable bowel syndrome, constipation, diarrhea, incontinence, GERD, and biliary disorders. Provides information on recent research.

Society of Gastroenterology Nurses and Associates, Inc.

www.sgna.org ****
Includes position statements, a discussion forum, certification information, scholarship information, a speakers bureau, and employment network, plus links to related sites.

GERONTOLOGICAL NURSING

Administration on Aging

www.aoa.dhhs.gov *****
Includes legislation related to aging, statistics about older people, and a resource directory for older adults. Also includes information for caregivers and elder abuse prevention, among many other items. Professional information includes legislation and program initiatives. Available in Spanish language.

Alzheimer's Association

www.alz.org *****
Contains information about the organization. Good information on signs and symptoms, treatment options, current research, and FAQs and expert answers. Also includes programs and resources and other Internet links. A poll is included on a timely topic.

Alzheimer's Disease Center

www.mayo.edu/research/alzheimers_center ***
Mayo Clinic center funded by the National Institutes for Health. Describes research areas and lists dementia classes and support groups. Provides information on risk factors, diagnosis, treatment, and caregiving strategies, as well as resources for professionals and the community.

Alzheimer's General Information Directory

www.alzforum.org/public/layperson_sites.html *****
Sponsored by the Alzheimer's Research Forum. Contains basic information on pathology, diagnosis, and treatment. Also an interactive Q&A page. Many links to good related sites such as those offering news about advances in research and treatment.

Alzheimer's Research Forum

www.alzforum.org/ ****
Includes a wide variety of information such as basic background on the disease, related Web sites, a list of Alzheimer's associations, a list of Alzheimer's disease centers, support and advocacy groups. Also includes information for researchers in the form of news, journal articles, discussion forums, and available jobs. There are treatment guides for physicians and a directory of drugs in clinical trials.

Gerontological Nursing Resources

www.uncg.edu/nur/gerohome.htm ***
Site of University of North Carolina, Greensboro. Very useful links to gerontological resources on the Web, including the U.S. Census Bureau, U.S. Administration on Aging, AARP, and the National Institute on Aging.

The Gerontological Society of America

www.geron.org ***
This organization's Web site includes conference information, a newsletter, contact points for interest groups, grant sources, and links to other sites on aging. Also lists publications and minority programs.

Medicare

medicare.gov *****
Information about the Medicare program, various health plans, and procedures for enrollment. Explains nursing homes and Medicare. Includes top 20 questions from the Medicare hotline, and information on fraud and abuse.

National Aging Information Center

www.aoa.dhhs.gov/NAIC/Notes/default.htm *****
Links to dozens of sites on aging, listed alphabetically by topics such as: adult day services, assisted living, case management, elder law, exercise and fitness, falls, grandparents raising grandchildren, mental health and aging, nursing homes, nutrition, and videos on aging.

National Osteoporosis Foundation

www.nof.org/osteoporosis ****
Basic information on osteoporosis, risk factors, causes, and prevalence. Information on bone density measures, prevention, and medications. Includes clinical guidelines for professionals and information on clinical conferences.

National Parkinson Foundation, Inc.

www.parkinson.org ****
Contains news, facts, resources, conferences, and clinical trials. Also has "tests" or questionnaires for Parkinson's, such as an anxiety scale, behavior tests, insomnia test, memory test, and so on. Also includes related links and a library.

GRANT SOURCES

American Nurses Foundation

www.ana.org/anf/nrggrant.htm ****
The ANF research grants program was founded over 40 years ago. Funded by donations from organizations and individuals. Lists recent award recipients, potential grant sources, and deadlines for applications. Only registered nurses with a baccalaureate or higher degree are eligible. Information packets are mailed.

The Foundation Center

fdncenter.org ****
A portal to grants available through private, corporate, and public foundations. You can search for foundations by name, by the top 100 foundations list, by the Grantmaker Web Sites, and by links to nonprofit resources. Includes online orientation for grantsmanship. *Note:* It is easiest to use this site by accessing the site map first.

GrantsNet

www.hhs.gov/grantsnet *****
Department of Health and Human Services site. Includes a "roadmap" to get you to DHHS grant information you want. Includes funding opportunities, the application process, how to write a grant, and how to manage a grant.

Health Resources and Services Administration

www.hrsa.dhhs.gov *****
Overview of this government agency and its grant programs. Grants are available from the Bureau of Primary Health Care, the Bureau of Health Professions, Bureau of Maternal and Child Health, and the HIV/AIDS Bureau. Grant cycles vary. Grant application guidance is available.

National Institutes of Health

grants.nih.gov/grants/index.cfm *****
The grants page gives information about applying for a grant or fellowship, administrative responsibilities of awardees, and peer review policies. Information about present and past awards can be accessed through the CRISP database link. Links to the Institutes of NIH give ideas about types of research areas of interest.

Robert Wood Johnson Foundation

www.rwjf.org/main.html ****
Contains information about the foundation, and a funding overview, with the amount of dollars spent in various project areas. Types of funding are: programs to reduce harm caused by substance abuse, programs to improve care for chronic health conditions, and programs to assure primary health care to all Americans. Information about current grants and how to apply for a grant are included.

HEALTH ASSESSMENT

Assessment—Interactive Health Evaluation

www.wehealnewyork.org/interactive/assessment.html **
A quick, general health appraisal with feedback. Fill out the questionnaire about demographics, medical history, and health habits, specific information for women or men, and you will get back a personalized health evaluation.

Auscultation—Virtual Stethoscope

www.music.mcgill.ca/auscultation/auscultation.html *****
Excellent tool for practice with heart and lung sounds. Includes normal and abnormal sounds with written descriptions. Diagrams show stethoscope placement. Requires sound card and speakers.

The Auscultation Assistant

www.med.ucla.edu/wilkes/Systolicbanner.htm ****
From UCLA Medical Center, audio files of a variety of heart murmurs and breath sounds with explanatory text. Includes information on normal sounds as well as abnormal. Includes information on the physiology of heart murmurs and some information on the conditions in which they occur.

Health Assessment

seniorhealth.about.com/seniorhealth/msubhealthassess.htm ****
A variety of personal health assessments, some of which are fun to do. Includes a "Hearing Test," "Lifestyle Inventory," "Longevity Assessment," and "Memory Quiz." Includes many good links including one on healthy living.

Heart Beats

www.medlib.com/spi/coolstuff2.htm ****
Contains audio files of normal and abnormal heart sounds. You must turn up your speakers to hear well. Heart sounds of common disease conditions are included. Also includes links to related sites.

Personal Assessments & Labs

www.mhhe.com/hper/health/personalhealth/labs *****
Part of McGraw-Hill publishing. The labs are a variety of assessment forms and measurements for personal health such as cardiovascular labs, chronic disease labs, nutrition labs, stress labs, substance abuse labs, and so on. Includes case studies. Blood pressure procedure is included.

The R.A.L.E. Repository

www.RALE.ca ***
Audio files and digital recordings of respiratory sounds, both normal and abnormal. Includes demonstration software for heart sounds. Information about products for sale is also included.

HISTORY OF NURSING

American Association for the History of Nursing, Inc.

www.aahn.org ****
Includes information about this professional organization plus a list of nursing history resources and archives. Also an interesting Gravesite feature picturing the gravesites of famous nurses along with their biographies. Includes a nice gift shop.

Black Nurses in History

www4.umdnj.edu/camlbweb/blacknurses.html ***
A good bibliography and guide to Web resources on historically significant black nurses, their contributions to the profession, and their struggle for equality. Also includes links to resources on the famous black nurses themselves.

Brownson's Nursing Notes

members.tripod.com/~DianneBrownson/ **
A simple but excellent list of links to resources for nursing history. Includes books, documents, and pictures of military nursing such as in the Civil War and the World Wars, as well as civilian nursing such as the Frontier Nursing Service.

Center for Nursing Historical Inquiry

www.nursing.virginia.edu/centers/cnhi.html ***
The Center is housed at the University of Virginia School of Nursing. The collection contains interesting photographs and descriptions of a large manuscript collection. The Center also runs a regular series of nursing history forums. Historical links are included.

Florence Nightingale Museum

www.florence-nightingale.co.uk ***
Details about the museum and its holdings are described. The Florence Nightingale story is told. Includes events and educational resources and services, and links to related organizations.

The Hall of Fame

www.ana.org/hof/index.htm ***
Includes a list of all inductees in the Nurses' Hall of Fame sponsored by the American Nurses Assocation, with links to their pictures and biographies.

Josephine A. Dolan Collection

www.cla.lib.ct.us/DoddCenter/ASC/nursing/dolan1.htm ***
Nursing history collection maintained by the University of Connecticut libraries and the Thomas Dodd Research Center. Includes a list of collection holding, including Civil War nursing, nursing organizations, nursing leaders, the Wolcott collection, and nursing education.

HOLISTIC NURSING (*SEE ALSO* ALTERNATIVE AND COMPLEMENTARY MEDICINE)

AHHA

www.ahha.org ****
Site of the American Holistic Health Association with explanation of its mission and history. Includes definition of holistic health, self-help articles, and databases of AHHA practitioner members. Also provides health information search services.

American Holistic Nurses Association

www.ahna.org ***
Organizational purpose, history, and membership information. Also includes educational opportunities, event notices, publications and products, and links to related sites.

HOSPICE

Hospice

dying.miningco.com/health/dying/cs/hospice/index.htm *****
Excellent resource for hospice information on topics like how to decide on whether to use a hospice, assessing functional status of the dying, cognitive disturbances during dying, and debunking myths about hospice.

Hospice Hands

hospice-cares.com **
Site sponsored by the North Central Florida Hospice. Includes basic information about hospice care and palliative care. Includes articles and book reviews, discussion groups, and information on employment. Includes links to related sites.

National Hospice Foundation

www.hospiceinfo.org/body.cfm ***
This is a charitable organization created to broaden understanding of hospice through research and education. Site includes a consumer's guide to selecting a hospice program, information on communicating your end-of-life wishes, Medicare hospice benefit, and description of the initiatives undertaken by the organization such as an HBO documentary and a photo exhibit.

National Hospice and Palliative Care Organization

www.nhpco.org/body.cfm ****
Basic information on hospice care. Information on conferences, and statistics on hospice care. Enables you to find local hospice programs.

Pam's Place on the Web

www.cp-tel.net/pamnorth/ ****
A great site for hospice resources but also for nurses and nursing students looking for an uncluttered site with a lot of helpful general interest sources of information. It makes the Web a source of inspiration for being a nurse and allows you to use the Internet to support both yourself and your patients.

HUMOR

All Nurses

allnurses.com ***
Click "Nursing Humor." A variety of nursing and medical jokes, cartoons, and funny stories—but many are one per page and some require linking to other sites.

American Association for Therapeutic Humor

www.aath.org ****
The association was created to educate health professionals and laypersons about the value of therapeutic humor. It serves as a clearinghouse of information on humor and laughter as they relate to well-being. Also includes an annotated bibliography on articles related to various aspects of humor and health.

International Center for Humor and Health

www.humorandhealth.com ****
A nonprofit organization whose purpose is to spread the healing art of laughter and to serve as a research center on humor and health. Programs include a National Clown and Laughter Hall of Fame; sending clowns to hospitals, nursing homes, and schools; and Humor and Health Management Workshops for businesses and educational settings. They also advertise a worldwide speakers bureau for keynote speeches or full-day seminars to help employees learn to utilize laughter to increase work satisfaction and productivity.

MC MD

members.aol.com/mcmdcomic/index.htm ***
Contains a biweekly comic strip poking gentle fun at the managed care industry. Strips are four panels and contain a managed care physician in the shape of a stethoscope. Strips go back to 1996.

Nurse Friendly

nursefriendly.com/nursing/humor/bedside.nursing.humor.htm ****
Several nursing jokes and stories like, "Harry Was in the Hospital" and "Urine Testing," and a large directory of humor-related sites.

Nurses Portal

www.virtualnurse.com/nursing/nursing-humor.html ***
A portal to many sites containing good jokes, stories, and cartoons related to health care, but lots of advertising.

Nurstoon

nurstoon.com *****
Site developed by an individual nurse. Very funny nurse-related cartoons and comic strips. Can send greeting cards and join a mailing list.

INFECTION CONTROL

CDC Division of Healthcare Quality Promotion

www.cdc.gov/ncidod/hip/default.htm *****
A wealth of information on infection control. Includes information about this branch of the Centers for Disease Control. Also the following topics: antimicrobial resistance, bloodborne pathogens, child care, dialysis, guidelines and recommendations, occupational health, outbreaks, sterilization and disinfection, and surveillance.

Infection Control

www.hopkins-id.edu/infcontrol/infection.html ****
Site developed by Johns Hopkins University. Includes infection control policies and procedures, isolation types, infection control practices, resistant organisms, outbreak investigations, and post-exposure prophylaxis. Infection control forms are also attached.

National Antimicrobial Information Network

ace.ace.orst.edu/info/nain ****
The site is a cooperative project of Oregon State University and the U.S. Environmental Protection Agency. Lists antimicrobial chemicals and gives fact sheets, safety guidelines, regulations, registration, toxicology, and other general information. Chemicals listed include alcohols, ethyline oxide, formaldehyde, hypochlorites, chlorine, and so on.

LISTSERVS AND NEWSGROUPS

Catalist

www.lsoft.com/catalist.html ***
The official catalogue of lists using the L-soft program. The site is intuitive with an internal search engine. It does not index lists using any other list distribution program, such as Majordomo or listproc.

Deja Newsgroups

groups.google.com *****
This premiere index of newsgroups was acquired in early 2001 by Google.com, a search engine company. The index will benefit from Google's expertise in organizing information. Expect Google's popularity to increase as well, as most nursing professional news-

groups reside in Europe. U.S. nurses primarily belong to listserv groups.

Nursing World e lists

www.ana.org/listserv/ ****
A very reliable source of listservs. A good place to start when selecting a nursing-related discussion group. The new subscriber will need assistance in determining the appropriate subscribing command for the administrative address provided.

Tile.Net

tile.net/lists/ ****
This comprehensive index of listservs is easy to use and offers searching by name, description, or domain. There is no way of telling how active a group may be except by the address that may indicate the listserv is part of a class or organization.

Topica

www.topica.com/ **
This index of discussion groups, newsgroups, and lists is geared for the public. It has an internal search engine but places it below linked categories of grouped mailing lists. Administrative addresses are not provided until after you have enrolled using the Topica interface.

MATERNAL–CHILD NURSING/MIDWIFERY

American College of Nurse Midwives

www.acnm.org ****
Includes information about the organization, standards of practice, code of ethics, and how to find a nurse midwife. Also includes information on continuing education, a bibliography, available jobs, and scholarships for nursing students. A bookstore is available.

AWHONN

www.awhonn.org ****
Information on the organization, continuing education, the convention, position statements, evidence-based practice guidelines, and legislative issues. Also includes a list of available jobs, an online store, and information on consulting services.

Baby Zone

www.babyzone.com *****
Useful information for pregnant women or those who want to adopt. Includes how to develop a birth plan, a due date calculator, help with baby names, adoption information, birth stories, e-cards, and a chat room.

Birthcenters

www.birthcenters.org/intro.shtml ****
Everything you wanted to know about Birth Centers—what they are, how to find one, and FAQs. Also includes a virtual tour of a birth center with audiovisual effects. Includes information about nurse midwifery, breaking news, and convention news.

Nurse Midwifery

www.nursefriendly.com/nursing/midwife.htm **
A portal to nurse midwifery and related sites. Includes a site for schools by state, midwife practitioner resources, labor and delivery sites, medication administration, and state-specific nurse midwife information.

MEDICAL CODING AND BILLING

eMDs

www.e-mds.com/icd9/index.html ***
A site with the International Classification of Diseases ICD-9 codes. You can search them by consecutive number or by number search. This list covers the entire list of official disease descriptions and their codes plus 50,000 alternate descriptions.

TDRweb

www.tdrdata.com/ICDCodeSearch.htm ***
Site of Timely Data Resources, a company providing information for pharmaceutical companies and health care professionals. You can search for International Classification of Disease by word, phrase, or by ICD-9 code number. You can also browse items by code groups.

MEDICATION CALCULATION

Basic Drug Calculation Review

www2.kumc.edu/instruction/nursing/n420/clinical/basic_review. htm *****
Site from University of Kansas. Review of common drug calculations with sample problems for nonparenteral, parenteral, and intravenous medications. Includes pediatric calculations and a list of additional practice sites. Includes ratio and proportion, desired/have formula, calculations based on units, and calculations based on weight.

Learning Laboratory

www.nursing.hhsweb.com/kuczek/310lab.htm ***
Sample medication problems and answers for an undergraduate course at Northern Illinois University (click on medication calculation test). Includes problems and tutorials on ratio and proportion, metric conversion, intravenous calculations, and fluid dosage calculations.

Medical Calculators

www-users.med.cornell.edu/~spon/picu/calc/medcalc.htm ****
From Weill Cornell Medical Center, NY. A very useful set of calculators for quick use. Includes calculators for emergency medication and drip rate-dose tables, and conversions for age, body surface area, calcium equivalents, temperature, length, weight, and pressure. Also metabolic calculators for body mass index, creatinine clearance, and serum osmolality.

Medication Calculation Work Sheet #1

www.ferris.edu/htmls/academics/course.offerings/hoisington denise/pharm151/math6.htm **
Tutorial on common drug calculations including conversions from metric to apothecary systems, dosage calculations, intravenous and IVPB calculations, and figuring concentrations.

Pharmacology Math

www.accd.edu/sac/nursing/math/mathindex.html ***
Practice quizzes on equivalencies, abbreviations, ratio and proportion, intravenous rates, and titration. Includes matching questions and multiple-choice questions. Feedback is provided on answers.

Weights and Measures

www.rxdesktop.com/weights_measures.htm **

Site sponsored by Taro Pharmaceuticals. This is a calculator for weight, fluid volume, and temperature conversion between metric, apothecary, and household systems that can be useful for quick conversions.

MENTAL HEALTH NURSING

APNA

www.apna.org *****

Site of the American Psychiatric Nurses Association. Organizational information, membership, headline news, conferences, legislation, job opportunities, and clinical information included. Also can access practice standards and videos and brochures that are available.

Center for Mental Health Services

www.mentalhealth.org ****

Part of the Knowledge Exchange Network of the U.S. Department of Health and Human Services. Description of the Center's mental health programs such as the child, adolescent, and family program, and the homelessness program. Also lists of mental health information such as consumer/survivor information, antistigma information, mental health parity, school violence prevention, and state resource guides. Available in Spanish language.

Internet Mental Health

www.mentalhealth.com/main.html *****

A wealth of information on mental health and illnesses. Includes descriptions of 54 common mental disorders with diagnosis, treatment, and research findings. Describes 72 common psychiatric drugs. Provides online assessment and diagnosis of problems like anxiety disorders, mood disorders, schizophrenia, eating disorders, and substance abuse disorders. Diagnosis is based on self-administered questionnaires and needs to be confirmed by a professional. Available in Spanish language.

NAMI

www.nami.org *****
Site of the National Alliance for the Mentally Ill, a grassroots advocacy organization. A wealth of information for lay people and professionals. Find out about the history of the organization, policy and legislative information, and "where we stand" position papers on mental health issues. Includes information for parents and links to sites on specific disorders.

MICROBIOLOGY

Introduction to Microbiology

www-micro.msb.le.ac.uk/109/BS109.html ***
From the United Kingdom, a course in basic microbiology. Lecture notes are on topics like history of microbiology, techniques, prokaryote diversity, environmental microbiology, and virus structures. Lecture notes include graphs, charts, and PowerPoint slides. Laboratory procedures requires a Quick Time plug-in.

Microbiology Webbed Out

www.bact.wisc.edu/microtextbook/TOC.html ***
From the University of Wisconsin—Madison, a microbiology textbook online. Textbook chapters include diagrams and charts. A topic search feature is available.

NCLEX REVIEW

National Council of State Boards of Nursing

www.ncsbn.org *****
Information about the NCLEX examination and the Candidate Diagnostic Profile. Includes an overview of the exam and how it is developed, test plans, FAQs about the exam, and rules for taking the exam. Also includes news bulletins about NCLEX and how professionals can participate in item development.

NursingNet

www.nursingnet.org/review.htm **
Links to four NCLEX review programs: EXAMCO, Kaplan's, NSNA EXCELL, and Sylvia Rayfield and Associates. More links are to be added as programs are reviewed.

NEUROLOGICAL NURSING

American Association of Neuroscience Nurses

www.aann.org ***
The Association is comprised of over 3,000 professionals dedicated to improving neuroscience health care. These professionals work in neurological units, rehabilitation units, neuropsychiatry, emergency departments, and many other clinical areas. The site includes information on membership, publications, educational resources, and a career advancement program. A bulletin board in also included.

American Stroke Association

www.strokeassociation.org *****
This organization is a division of the American Heart Association. The site includes warning signs of stroke, risk assessment, and stroke prevention and treatment. The Heart and Stroke A–Z Guide includes an alphabetical listing of biostatistical fact sheets that are very informative.

National Stroke Association

www.stroke.org/index.cfm *****
A wonderful resource on stroke and TIA. Includes prevention, treatment, and rehabilitation information. Also has survivor and caregiver information, prevention programs, and professional products such as the NIH Stroke Scale Exam, a Risk Disk, and many pamphlets and slide shows.

Traumatic Brain Injury Resource Guide

www.neuroskills.com *****
Wonderful resource for traumatic brain injury pathology, and coma and vegetative states. Includes links to assessment scales such as Glasgow Coma Scale and Disability Rating Scale. Research on nerve regeneration is described.

NURSE PRACTITIONERS

American Academy of Nurse Practitioners

www.aanp.org ***
Contains information on the organization, current news, conferences, legislative and regulatory information, position statements,

and a list of Fellows of the Academy. Certification information is included. Tips on developing contracts and practice agreements are included.

Internet Resources for Nurse Practitioner Students

nurseweb.ucsf.edu/www/arwwebpg.htm ***
Developed by an NP graduate of the University of California, San Francisco. A series of links to sites that would be helpful to NP students. Categories are: Health Information Gateways, Nurse Practitioner/Nursing Resources, Clinical Practice Guidelines, Primary Care, Pediatrics, Adolescent Health, School-Based Health Care, and Women's Health. Last updated in 1999.

Medscape Nursing—Ask the Experts

www.medscape.com/Home/network/nursing/directories/dir NURS.AskExperts.html ***
This service allows nurse practitioners to submit questions from a panel of experts. Questions should be on clinical topics, but not a specific consultation on an individual patient. Approximately two per week are submitted to the experts. Recent discussions have been on topics like legal issues, cardiology, diabetes, and other specialties. Examples of questions are: "How does a leased employee agreement work?" "What is my obligation to provide care for individuals who are not my clients?" and "Can I perform advanced procedures I have been trained for without a physician present?"

National Organization of Nurse Practitioner Faculties

www.nonpf.com ****
Organization provides leadership in promoting quality nurse practitioner education. Site includes membership information, current news, conferences, and publications. Links to other nursing organizations are included.

NURSING LANGUAGES

Alternative Link

www.alternativelink.com ****
The site provides samples of applications and links to the vendor of CAM-Net MIS. A data set based on coded procedures for Com-

plementary and Alternative Medicine (CAM) and nursing. The data set distinguishes itself by providing coding for alternative practice areas such as chiropractic, acupuncture, homeopathy, nurse midwife, and licensed practical nurses.

ANA Recognized Languages for Nursing

nursingworld.org/nidsec/nilang.htm ****
The home page of the Nursing Information Data Set Evaluation Center (NIDSEC) is the best place to start on the Web in a study of nursing languages. This list is limited to American data sets, however. There are links to the approved data sets Web pages or to the author's e-mail.

Health Level Seven

www.hl7.org/ ****
Health Level Seven (HL7) is the premiere standard setting organization for the exchange of data that supports clinical patient care and management. The organization studies linkages of data and sets standards that facilitate exchange across different platforms of health care information systems.

Home Health Care Classification System

www.sabacare.com/ ****
A clear, intuitive, yet simple, Web page about a nursing language or classification system. Dr. Virginia Saba shares the system she has developed and tested at Georgetown University including links to others who have contributed to the literature about the HHCC system. HHCC was one of the first four nursing classification systems approved by NICSEC of the American Nurses Association.

International Classification for Nursing Practice

icn.ch/icnp.htm ****
The International Council of Nurses has developed the ICNP®. It provides a unifying framework into which existing nursing vocabularies can be cross-mapped to enable comparison of nursing data collected using other recognized nursing vocabularies and classifications.

NIC and NOC

www.nursing.uiowa.edu/cnc/index.htm ****
The Center for Nursing Classification at the University of Iowa has developed two nursing languages known as Nursing Interventions Classification (NIC) system and Nursing Outcomes Classification (NOC) system. These NICSEC approved classifications are very comprehensive vocabulary networks. Links to resources and use permits for the classifications are available.

North American Nursing Diagnosis Association

www.nanda.org/ **
Everyone associated with nursing is aware of the approved list of Nursing Diagnoses that are published biannually, so this site would be an easy find using your Web browser. Unfortunately, all that is found is an order form to obtain the list. Disappointing.

OMAHA

con.ufl.edu/Omaha *
The Omaha nursing classification system was one of the first four approved by NIDSEC. This is the designated Web site but it offers little information about the system. The Omaha system is the reference system used in the FITNE Nightingale Tracker but the link was broken when clicked. The site needs to be updated.

Perioperative Nursing Data Set

www.aorn.org/research/pnds.htm **
The Perioperative Nursing Data Set (PNDS) is a nursing language system developed by and for perioperative nurses. Endorsed by NICSEC in 1999, the framework is described but specifics are not available here.

SNOMED RT

www.snomed.org *****
This informative Web site describes the Systematized Nomenclature of Medicine Reference Terminology (SNOMED RT) developed to gather detailed clinical information. The vocabulary is recognized and used globally. This terminology is designed to index the entire health care record and not merely nursing, medicine, billing, and so on. The site is the most informative of the nursing language or classification system Web sites.

NURSING THEORY

Nursing Theory Link Page

healthsci.clayton.edu/eichelberger/nursing.htm *****
Authored by Clayton College and State University, Department of
Nursing. Contains links to all major nursing theorist sites as well
as some lesser-known theorists. Also contains a reference list and
advice for searching nursing theory references.

Nursing Theory Page

www.ualberta.ca/~jrnorris/nt/theory.html *****
Contains a link or series of links to all major nursing theorist Web
pages. Also links to lesser-known nursing theories and related
health care theories. Includes literature search tips, references, and
information about upcoming theorist conferences.

NUTRITION

Botanical.com — A Modern Herbal

www.botanical.com/botanical/mgmh/comindxe.html ***
An index of modern herbs listed by common names. Search alphabetically for the herb you are interested in. For each herb, there is
a description, constituents, other names, and medicinal uses. Site
also includes an index of recipes and index of poisons.

Center for Food Safety & Applied Nutrition

vm.cfsan.fda.gov/list.html *****
A Center of the Food and Drug Administration. Includes FDA regulations on specified topics, information on FDA projects and programs. Contains information on dietary supplements, foodborne
illnesses, food labeling, and food additives. Lists available videos.

Cook's Thesaurus

www.foodsubs.com ***
A cooking encyclopedia covering thousands of ingredients. Includes pictures, descriptions, pronunciations, and suggested sub-
stitutions for cooking. Major categories include vegetables, fruits,
dairy, liquids, grains, baked goods, meats, fish, vegetarian, baking
supplies, condiments, and equipment.

Cyberdiet

www.cyberdiet.com ****
The site was developed by two individuals with a community advisory board. Information is peer reviewed. Contains a great deal of useful information on diets, weight loss, eating right, dining out, vitamins, exercise, pregnancy, and diabetic diets. Also includes some nice assessment tools, a discussion group, and an Ask the Expert feature.

Nutrient Data Laboratory

www.nal.usda.gov/fnic/cgi-bin/nut_search.pl ***
Search the USDA Nutrient Database to find all nutritional values of foods. Enter your food name, for example, "ice cream," and you will obtain a list of foods containing ice cream. Select the particular food product and you will get a list of the minerals, vitamins, lipids, carbohydrates, proteins, fiber, and calories in that food. Loading is slow.

Pediatric Nutrition

pediatrics.about.com/health/pediatrics/cs/nutrition/index.htm ****
A portal through About.com to a variety of sites about pediatric nutrition. Find out what is the best to feed infants, children, and teenagers. Links are available to "Nutrition and Fitness for Kids" and "LaLeche League."

ONCOLOGY NURSING

American Cancer Society

www.cancer.org *****
Information on types of cancer, prevention, and information resources for people with cancer, including complementary and alternative methods. Helpful information for cancer nurse researchers, including some questionnaires. Bookstore available. Some information also in Spanish.

Association of Cancer Online Resources (ACOR)

www.acor.org/index.html ***
A portal for a variety of unique Web sites and electronic mailing lists, which are online support groups for specific types of cancer

like bladder cancer, breast cancer, lymphoma, and so on. Also includes a searchable database of news articles about cancer.

Cancerlinks

www.cancerlinks.org *****
Wonderful resources of extensive links to sites on specific carcinomas, with a wide variety of information on each. For example, Bladder Cancer links include general medical information, treatment, journals, quackery, and clinical trials. Contains a tutorial on searching the Web.

Cancer Nursing Education

profed.uicc.org/nurses ***
Information on international courses in oncology nursing. Includes a few links to cancer sites and articles, as well as the history and mission of the organization.

Oncolink

cancer.med.upenn.edu ****
A series of links to links. Includes many great resources regarding specific cancers, symptom management, cancer causes, clinical trials, global resources, and FAQs. Also addresses financial issues for patients.

ONS online

www.ons.org **
Site of the Oncology Nursing Society. Requires that you register (free) in order to obtain information either for health care providers or consumers. Includes information on conferences, the organization itself, clinical practice, education, and a library.

ONLINE JOURNALS

Advance for Nurses

www.ADVANCEforNurses.com/ ****
An online and print journal designed to address regional issues as well as offer continuing education opportunities. It is not peer reviewed. There are currently four regional issues, all in the eastern seaboard of the United States.

Free Medical Journals

www.freemedicaljournals.com/ ****
This site is dedicated to providing free access to medical journals. It has a global flavor as evidenced by its sort feature of articles and journals in English, French, Spanish, Portuguese, and a number of other languages.

Harden MD (Free full text medical/nursing journals)

www.lib.uiowa.edu/hardin/md/ej.html *****
A comprehensive collection of medical and other health care related journals for which there are full-text, free access to users of the Internet. Most of the journals are print journals and not technically online journals.

Information Technology in Nursing

www.bcsnsg.org.uk/itin/ *****
Information Technology in Nursing (ITIN) is the official journal of the Nursing Specialist Group of The British Computer Society. The Web site offers links to the news items of issues in PDF format but not full text of the articles. Its focus is on nursing informatics in the United Kingdom and Europe.

Internet Scientific Publications

www.ispub.com/journals/ija.htm ***
This is an index of Scientific Ejournals. The membership is free and allows the user to receive e-mails on a variety of information including FDA alerts. Most journals were medical specialty specific. One new addition contains articles for nonprofessionals about health and health care.

Journal of American Medical Informatics Association

www.jamia.org/ *****
JAMIA is the bimonthly journal of the American Medical Informatics Association published since 1994. It is a print journal of peer reviewed articles on health care informatics that is available online by subscription. The abstracts can be browsed for free. Full text requires membership.

The Journal of Clinical Investigation

www.jci.org/ ***
This journal of clinical research reports is published online by Stanford University. The site provides abstracts and full text of all journal issues dating back to January 1997. A very intuitive site.

Journal of Undergraduate Nursing Scholarship

www.juns.nursing.arizona.edu/ ****
Founded in 1999, the full-text articles represent some of the wonderful writing produced by baccalaureate nursing students. The journal is sure to flourish as information seeking via the Internet becomes ubiquitous.

MMWR Weekly

www.cdc.gov/mmwr//mmwr_wk.html ****
The Morbidity and Mortality Weekly Report from the Centers for Disease Control and Prevention (CDC) can be downloaded via PDF file from this site. An important journal for public health nurses, the online format makes storage and searching easier than traditional bookshelves.

Online Journal of Nursing Informatics

www.hhdev.psu.edu/nurs/ojni/index.htm ****
The first online peer reviewed journal for nurses, it was launched in December of 1996. Archives contain six past issues and articles are available free. It is indexed in CINAHL. The site is easy to navigate.

ORTHOPEDICS

About Orthopedics

orthopedics.about.com/health/orthopedics/mbody.htm *****
Portal to many sites related to orthopedic conditions. For example, sites on sprains and strains, broken bones, arthroscopy, arthritis, osteoporosis, and tumors. Also gives answers to FAQs about orthopedic problems and suggestions on how to find an orthopedic surgeon.

National Association of Orthopaedic Nursing

naon.inurse.com ****
Web site of the association. Includes information on the organization, certification in orthopedic nursing, and continuing education. Also has an online forum for discussions, legislative information, news, and available grants and awards.

Orthopedics & Bone Diseases

www.lib.uiowa.edu/hardin/md/ortho.html *****
University of Iowa site. Portal to many sites related to orthopedics. Includes links to MEDLINE and disease-specific sites with information on pathology, treatment, and clinical trials. Includes adult and pediatric sites.

PAIN

American Academy of Pain Management

www.aapainmanage.org ****
Information about the organization and a membership directory. Also includes basic information like the Patients' Bill of Rights, finding a pain management program, and FAQs for patients and doctors. The National Pain Data Bank is the Academy's outcomes measurement database to see the results of specific treatments for specific conditions.

Hospice Net: Pain Control

www.hospicenet.org/html/pain_myths.html ****
Explains and debunks common myths about pain control in hospice patients, such as "People who take Morphine will become addicted," and "People who take Morphine will die sooner because Morphine causes them to stop breathing."

PAIN

adultpain.nursing.uiowa.edu/ *****
A premiere site on the Internet for nursing interested in pain assessment and management for all ages. The University of Iowa College of Nursing has received federal funds to develop and support this frequently visited site. I would recommend the site to patients.

Pain Control After Surgery

my.webmd.com/content/dmk/dmk_article_51980 ****
Good resource (basically a pamphlet) for laypersons on methods
of pain control after surgery. Discussion of goals of pain control
and types of treatment. Drug treatment and nondrug treatment
are discussed. Based on AHCPR guidelines.

PainLink

www.edc.org/PainLink/index.html *****
Many free resources such as clinical practice guidelines on management of varied types of pain, use of placebos, use of opioids for chronic
pain, and so on. Also includes a case study and quiz. Institutions may
join the organization with a fee and access further resources.

Palliative Care Resource Center

mayday.coh.org/_private/home.htm ***
The City of Hope Pain/Palliative Care site supported by Knoll
Pharmaceutical. Includes a list of topics like pain and quality of
life, pain in the elderly, pain in pediatrics, home care, pain and the
family, costs of pain management, and pharmacology.

Questions and Answers About Pain Control

cancernet.nci.nih.gov/peb/pain_control *****
Information for cancer patients and families regarding pain and its
relief. Sponsored by the American Cancer Society and National
Cancer Institute. Includes topics like What Is Pain, How to Relieve
Pain with Medicines, Nonprescription Pain Relievers, and Other
Methods of Pain Relief.

TNEEL (Toolkit for Nursing Excellence at End of Life Transition)

www.son.washington.edu/departments/bnhs/pain/index.html ***
The Cancer Pain and Symptom Management Nursing Research
Group (CPSMNRG) have created this site. The goal of these nurse
scientists and researchers is to generate and disseminate knowledge related to the pain and other symptoms experienced by people living with cancer and by people facing the end of life transi-
tion. Go here to access TNEEL, an interactive set of learning
modules appropriate for students and practicing nurses.

PATHOPHYSIOLOGY

Anemia

www.neosoft.com/~uthman/anemia/anemia.html ***
Excellent and comprehensive information on all types of anemias. Includes definitions, diagnosis, and some pictures and diagrams. However, there is a lot of text to read, and there is no indication of the date of the data.

Bone and Joint Pathology Index

www-medlib.med.utah.edu/WebPath/BONEHTML/BONEIDX. html ***
University of Utah medical library site. Good tutorial on osteoporosis with graph and references. Tissue images are given for many orthopedic conditions such as osteosarcoma, chondrosarcoma, Ewing's sarcoma, and metastatic carcinoma.

Cardiovascular Diseases

web.bu.edu/COHIS/cardvasc/cvd.htm ****
Wonderful basic information on cardiovascular pathophysiology. Includes information on blood problems, blood vessel problems, and heart problems (MI, CHF, cardiomyopathy, pericarditis, congenital disorders). Also includes information on risk factors, prevention, and diagnosis. Useful for nursing students and the lay public.

Central Nervous System Infections

edcenter.med.cornell.edu/Pathophysiology_Cases/CNS/CNS_TOCs .html **
Site of Cornell University Weill Medical College. Includes 14 cases with central nervous system infections. Each case includes a history and physical, MRI and CAT scans, and a list of questions followed by the answers.

Diagnosis and Pathophysiology of Osteoarthritis

www.ama-assn.org/med-sci/course/oa/diag.htm ***
Sponsored by the American Medical Association for Continuing Medical Education. Includes pathophysiology, diagnosis, classifications, and treatment of osteoarthritis. Especially focuses on the hip and knee.

Digital Slice of Life

www.medlib.med.utah.edu/kw/sol/sss *****
From the University of Utah medical library. Great digital images and tissue slides for learning pathology (and anatomy). Covers most body systems and will be expanding soon.

Drug Abuse Pathophysiology

www.nida.nih.gov/Diagnosis-Treatment/Diagnosis4.html ***
From the National Institute on Drug Abuse (NIH). Good information and references on the pathology of addiction, and assessment, diagnosis, and treatment of drug abuse. Some pictures and diagrams included.

HealthWeb

healthweb.org *****
Portal to pathophysiologic information on many disease conditions, listed alphabetically. For example, if you click Endocrinology, you can visit dozens of sites from universities and professional organizations that will review pathology, show tissue slides, give clinical guidelines, and position statements.

Lower Respiratory Tract Infections

edcenter.med.cornell.edu/Pathophysiology_Cases/Pulmonary/Pulm_TOCs.html ***
Cornell University Weill Medical College site. Includes 37 cases with lower respiratory tract infections. Each case includes a history and physical, chest x-rays or CAT scans, and a list of questions followed by the answers.

Pathology Online

www.pathoplus.com/ ****
Developed by a very Web-savvy nursing professor, Ken Zwolski. The site has many resources for learning about some basics, as well as concepts related to nursing and patient care. Go to the archives page for a full listing of the many topics available. Includes classic lectures and good links to nursing and health sites.

Pathophysiology of Asthma

www.ama-assn.org/med-sci/course/asthma/pathopsy.htm ****
Sponsored by the American Medical Association for Continuing Medical Education. Contains a comprehensive explanation of asthma, some case studies, classifications of asthma, and treatment regimens (step therapy and proactive maintenance therapy).

Pathophysiology of the Endocrine System

arbl.cvmbs.colostate.edu/hbooks/pathphys/endocrine ****
A project of Colorado State University to provide textbook-type course material on the Web. Excellent information on endocrine glands and hormones. Also includes information on regulatory processes like fuel metabolism, calcium homeostasis, and regulation of body weight. Some pictures and diagrams.

Pathophysiology of Infectious Diseases

www.courses.ahc.umn.edu/medical-school/IDis/class.html ****
University of Michigan Medical School site. Wonderful review of infectious disease processes in general, and a couple of specific disease entities. In addition, selected topics are: antibiotics, infections in the elderly, nosocomial infections, and septic shock. Good photographs and a multiple-choice examination. Last updated in 1997.

PEDIATRICS

General Pediatrics

generalpediatrics.com *****
Web portal to sites including case studies and patient simulations, evidence-based practice, policy statements and clinical practice guidelines, and professional organizations. Click on information for professionals or patients on about 200 common pediatric health problems.

Immunize for Healthy Lives

www.mcdonalds.com/countries/usa/community/health/index. html ****
The site was developed for a project called Immunize for Healthy Lives sponsored by the American Academy of Pediatrics (AAP), McDonald's® Restaurants, the National Association of County & City Health Officials (NACCHO), and the Blue Cross and Blue

Shield Association to educate people about the benefits of immunizations. Contains a wonderful printable immunization schedule. No in-depth discussion about the diseases that are prevented by the immunizations.

Mom's Refuge

www.momsrefuge.com/pediatrics ***
An interesting site on parenting, especially focused on working mothers. Contains a health newsletter written by a physician. Also information on Practical Parenting, Single Moms, Sports Mom, and the Art of Juggling. Includes a discussion list and business directory.

National Association of Pediatric Nurse Associates and Practitioners

www.napnap.org ****
Information about NAPNAP including membership information. Includes legislative news, job connections, grants, conference information, and pediatric-related links.

National Clearinghouse on Child Abuse and Neglect Information

www.calib.com/nccanch *****
The Clearinghouse is a national resource for professionals seeking information on the prevention, identification, and treatment of child abuse and neglect. Includes news, publications, potential funding sources, and databases. Also includes links to related sites.

Neonatal Nursing

www.nursingnet.org/neonurse/neonatal.htm ***
Topics listed are Clinical Information, Breastfeeding, Developmental Care, Infections, Neonatal Death/SIDS, Journals/Discussion Groups, Associations & Education, Parent Info Sites, and Advanced Technology. Includes many links in each topic.

Otitis Media

sibyl.uchsc.edu/vc/ear/index.cfm ****
The University of Colorado Health Science Center maintains this site. For students or nurses interested in the diagnosis and treat-

ment of Otitis Media, this site is fabulous. It is interactive, that is, you enter a response to get feedback about the appropriateness of the response. Check out the Pneumatic Otoscopy Review Course.

Pediatric Database

www.icondata.com/health/pedbase/index.htm ****
An alphabetical list of pediatric disorders. Each includes an outline of definition pathogenesis, clinical features, diagnosis, and management.

Pediatric Nursing News and Resources

www.pediatricnursing.com *****
Source of lots of information on news about various disease conditions, 120 case studies with x-rays, FAQs about becoming a pediatric nurse, and job listings. Links to other resources such as poison control centers and online drug reference.

Pediatrics

www.pediatrics.about.com/health/pediatrics/cs/diseaseac/index. htm *****
Web portal to a world of sites related to pediatrics. Subjects (links) include an alphabetical list of diseases, genetics, growth and development, health and safety, medications, nutrition, parenting, professional associations, special needs kids, health insurance, and well-child visits.

Pediatrics

dir.yahoo.com/Health/Medicine/Pediatrics ***
Directory through Yahoo.com leads to a wide variety of pediatric-related sites, including sites on pathology; pediatric critical care, orthopedics, infectious diseases, rheumatology, and cardiac arrest; pediatric organizations; pediatric database; neonatology network; and listservs.

PEDINFO

pedinfo.org/Nursing.html **
A list of links to pediatric nursing organizations and journals. Also contains a list of pediatric diseases and conditions with a Search feature. Some links are not active.

PERIOPERATIVE NURSING

Anesthesia Patient Safety

www.anesthesiapatientsafety.com ****
Web site designed to promote safe anesthesia patient care through public education. Includes content about anesthesia, medication complications, and conscious sedation. Includes a video "Best Kept Secret in Healthcare, About Nurse Anesthetists."

AORN Online

www.aorn.org ****
Site of the Association of periOperative Registered Nurses. Click on news, job database, bookstore, continuing education, AORN journal, specialty assemblies, and clinical practice. Includes FAQs on clinical issues like aseptic technique, counts, latex allergy, procedural sedation, skin prep, and so on.

Certification Board Perioperative Nursing

www.certboard.org ***
CNOR and CRNFA certification exams are listed. Applications available online. Objectives and purposes of certification are given. Information about preparatory courses for certification exams.

PHARMACOLOGY

Pharmacy On-Line

www.priory.com/pharmol.htm **
From the International Journal of Pharmacy, this site includes new drugs and those currently in the news. Click the drug topic of interest. There is also an Ask the Doctor feature, although not all questions that are submitted are answered.

PharmInfoNet

pharminfo.com *****
Very useful site on common diseases and drug therapy. Includes diseases and conditions like AIDS, asthma, cancer, cardiovascular, diabetes, respiratory, endocrine, hypertension, mental health, obesity, arthritis, and ulcers. Also includes discussion groups that are moderated by experts.

PharmWeb

www.pharmweb.net *****
Broad range of information on pharmacology. Resources available are discussion groups, chat rooms, newsgroups, a virtual library, patient information, government regulation, continuing education, and others.

PROFESSIONAL ORGANIZATIONS (OTHER THAN THE ONES LISTED UNDER SPECIALTY TOPICS)

American Association of Pediatrics

www.aap.org/ ***
The American Association of Pediatrics site is not just for physicians. It is directed toward pediatric residents and fellows but also outlines local conferences and research reports. There are links to Medline via Medscape. The site is searchable.

American Diabetes Association

www.diabetes.org *****
Overview of the ADA and general information on diabetes and management through nutrition and exercise. Includes clinical practice recommendations and information on current research. Also contains links to courses and continuing education programs for professionals. The recipe of the day and virtual grocery store are nice touches.

American Nurses Association

www.ana.org *****
Contains membership information, news in the nursing world, and information about ANA's programs such as the American Nurses Credentialing Center, the American Academy of Nursing, the American Nurses Foundation, and American Nurses Publishing. Also includes online continuing education offerings and information about international nursing.

American Public Health Association

www.apha.org *****
For 125 years, APHA has been setting public health priorities and influencing policies. The site contains information about the orga-

nization, a news room, publications, and job opportunities. Also included is a description of current programs, a list of state public health associations, and many related links to other sites.

American Red Cross

www.redcross.org *****
Lists and describes all Red Cross services such as Armed Forces Emergency Services, Biomedical Services, Disaster Services, Health and Safety Services, International Services, and Nursing. Explains how nurses and student nurses can get involved. You can locate your local Red Cross office.

Centers for Disease Control and Prevention

www.cdc.gov *****
Information about the organization, its mission, and its structure. Includes health topics and diseases listed alphabetically and data and statistics on health and disease. Traveler's information includes health information on specific destinations, vaccinations, diseases that can affect travelers, and traveling with children. Available in Spanish language.

Food and Drug Administration

www.fda.gov *****
Information on the products that the FDA regulates (food, drugs, medical devices, biologics, animal feed and drugs, cosmetics, and radiation-emitting products). Contains information for professionals and consumers. Opportunity to report (online) a problem with a product and to give your views on proposed FDA regulations. Links are provided to FDA manuals and publications.

International Council of Nurses

www.icn.ch *****
Includes information about the organization and its policies and programs. There is a newsroom and a bookstore. Nursing Matters fact sheets provide international perspectives on current health and social issues like birth registration, displaced persons, the health of indigenous peoples, poverty and health, and healthy ageing. Available in French and Spanish language.

National Institute of Nursing Research

www.nih.gov/ninr ****
The mission and history of the Institute are explained. Highlights research funding and programs such as traditional research grants and AREA grants. Currently funded projects are listed, as are research priority areas. Also includes publications available and FAQs.

National Institutes of Health

www.nih.gov *****
Overview of the NIH and its offices and programs. Links are available to NIH Institutes and Centers. Scientific resources include CancerNet (fact sheets on cancer), Consensus Statements (guides to current medical issues), and Grants Information. Clinical trial information, publications, and fact sheets are also provided. Available in Spanish language.

National Nursing Staff Development Organization

www.nnsdo.org/ ***
This is the home page of the National Nursing Staff Development Organization. It provides resources specific for agency education trends and strategies. A discussion forum is available to communicate with others of similar interest and needs. The site is simple with "few bells and whistles" but a necessity for in-service faculty and directors.

Sigma Theta Tau

www.nursingsociety.org *****
Contains information about STT, membership, news in the organization, and member surveys. Also information about awards and global opportunities. Continuing education case study offerings are available.

World Health Organization

www.who.int *****
Includes information about WHO and details some of its programs (e.g., AIDS and vaccines). Also has a database of communicable and infectious diseases listed alphabetically, and statistical data-

bases. The Weekly Epidemiological Report is available, providing timely epidemiological information and details of emerging disease outbreaks. Includes health topics like "health technology," "vaccine preventable diseases," and "family and reproductive health."

REHABILITATIVE NURSING

Association of Rehabilitation Nurses

www.rehabnurse.org ***
Membership and certification information included. Also includes grants available, job listings, conferences, online continuing education, and a listserv.

Spinal Cord Injury Information Network

www.spinalcord.uab.edu *****
Site from University of Alabama. Useful information on spinal cord injury rehabilitation, including occupational therapy, physical therapy, and therapeutic recreation. Also references equipment used in rehabilitation and rehab centers. The site also includes publications and links to disability organizations.

RESPIRATORY NURSING

American Lung Association

www.lungusa.org *****
Great source of information on respiratory diseases including AIDS-related lung disorders, asthma, bronchitis, COPD, lung cancer, and so on. Also has many printable information sheets on these conditions. Information on tobacco legislation and information on research awards and grants is included.

JAMA Asthma Information Center

www.ama-assn.org/special/asthma/treatmnt/treatmnt.htm ****
The Asthma Information Center of the Journal of the American Medical Association. Features a Treatment Center with clinical guidelines, treatment updates based on research such as, "Asthma and GERD," "Asthma and Pregnancy," "Asthma and Sinusitis," and "Inhaled Corticosteroids." Also includes a library.

SCHOOL NURSING

ASHA

www.ashaweb.org **
Site of the American School Health Association. Includes information on the organization, publications, conferences, and membership. Also available is an online membership application and scholarship application.

Healthy Schools Network

www.hsnet.org ***
This is a nonprofit organization dedicated to creating schools that are environmentally responsible to children and personnel. Includes an information clearinghouse with policy guides and information packets on school health topics like asbestos hazards, allergies and chemical sensitivities, air quality, and injury and fire safety.

National Assembly on School-Based Health Care

www.nasbhc.org ***
The organization is dedicated to providing school-based primary health care and mental health care for children through collaborative efforts. Nice information about school-based health centers, standards and guidelines for them, statistics, financing them, and evaluating them. Also includes information and links on school-based prevention programs.

STATISTICAL CONCEPTS AND CALCULATIONS

Electronic Textbook *Statsoft*

www.statsoft.com/textbook/esc1.html ****
An online statistics textbook that may be downloaded free to your hard drive. The textbook begins with basic statistical concepts, followed by groups of statistical techniques, organized into modules, accessible by buttons, representing classes of analytic techniques.

Rice Virtual Lab in Statistics

www.ruf.rice.edu/~lane/rvls.html *****
Contains online textbook *Hyperstat*. Also features simulations that are Java applets demonstrating various statistical concepts. There

are case studies with real data that is analyzed and interpreted and an analysis lab with some basic statistical tools.

Statistics Every Writer Should Know

www.robertniles.com/stats ***

Tutorial on basic statistical concepts. Very basic statistical concepts for novices, and frequently asked questions. Includes the "Stats Board" for posting your questions about statistics, or helping someone else with their question.

Web Pages That Perform Statistical Calculations

users.aol.com/johnp71/javastat.html ****

Contains links to many sites for free statistical calculations as well as sites that produce graphs and charts, for a total of 550 links. Some sites are tutorials on statistical tests or downloadable software and related resources. Not all links are active.

TELEHEALTH

Office for the Advancement of Telehealth

telehealth.hrsa.gov ****

Sponsored by the U.S. Health Resources and Services Administration. The office is designed to lead, coordinate, and promote telehealth technologies. Includes information on grants, services, and links to other sites.

UROLOGY

The Kidney Patient's Guide

www.kidneypatientguide.org.uk/site/HD.html *****

Great site. The home page states the site is "for kidney patients and the people who care for them." Contains several animations that facilitate the text explanations of the processes of renal structure, function, and effects of dysfunction. Also includes explanations about how an arteriovenous fistula is constructed and used in hemodialysis as well as the hemodialysis and peritoneal dialysis procedures.

Urologic Oncology Program

www.cancer.med.umich.edu/prostcan/prostcan.html ****
University of Michigan site contains up-to-date information on prostate cancer. Includes basic review, staging information, clinical trials at various sites, and information on videos available.

Urology

urology.medscape.com/Home/Topics/urology/urology.html ****
Web portal (Medscape) with a broad array of links to topics like "Today's Urology News," "Conference Summaries," "Resource Centers," "Library," "Journal Room," and a "Treatment Center."

Urology

dir.yahoo.com/Health/Medicine/Urology ***
Web portal (Yahoo) with a list of links to common urological disorders and their pathology and treatment. Information is given for professionals and lay people. There are links to related sites like uroradiology, exstrophy, and prostate cancer.

WOMEN'S HEALTH

Certified Mammography Facilities

www.fda.gov/cdrh/mammography/certified.html ***
A list of certified facilities, updated weekly. Click the Search link and access a listing by state and zip code of all facilities that meet baseline quality standards for equipment, personnel, and practices.

Contraception Information Center

www.ama-assn.org/special/contra/contra.htm ****
Produced by the Journal of the American Medical Association, this site is designed as a resource for health professionals. Provides links to patient education materials from Planned Parenthood, like "Your Contraceptive Choices," "The Condom," "Norplant and You," and "All about Vasectomy." Includes FAQs about contraception, and a library with abstracts of major articles on contraception, and some full-text articles.

Menopause Resource Guide

www.4woman.gov/owh/pub/menoguide.htm ****
A portal for links to government agencies, organizations, newsletters, books, magazines, and reports related to menopause. Includes full citations and addresses or phone numbers.

National Women's Health Information Center

www.4woman.gov *****
Health information and referral center for women, sponsored by the U.S. Department of Health and Human Services. Focus on news in women's health with press releases, and hot topics in Congress. Includes information on health pregnancy, breastfeeding, women with disabilities, violence against women, body image, and minority health information. Available in Spanish language.

WOUND CARE

Chronic Wound Healing

coninfo.nursing.UIOWA.EDU/sites/ChronicWound **
From the College of Nursing at University of Iowa. A brief tutorial on various aspects of wound care for health professionals. Includes definitions and descriptions, assessment, debridement, cleansing, maintaining a moist environment, support surfaces, and nutrition.

Wound Care Guide

www.bertek.com/burnandwound/woundcare.html **
Site developed by Bertek Pharmaceuticals Burn and Wound Products. Contains photographs of wounds at stages 1 through 4 and a skin tear and wound with eschar. Each photograph can be enlarged. Also includes case studies that explain how their wound care products are applied and are effective.

MISCELLANEOUS SITES

All Nurses

allnurses.com/ ****
This site has the look and feel of a commercial Web site. It is a commercial Web site but it offers a wide variety of topics of inter-

est to nurses and to student nurses as a one-stop-shopping site. A nice feature is the question at the bottom of the page that lets you vote on a question or issue and then see a report of all of the responses. Try it, it is fun and there are also links to nursing discussion lists, state boards of nursing, and nursing literature, to name a few.

Disability Information for Students

www.abilityinfo.com/ **
Offers information related to students with disabilities, but also many resources for parents of children with special needs. Has discussion forums and a chat room as well as references for sale and an international newswatch for disability information. Includes many links.

International Biometrics Group

www.biometricgroup.com/ ****
This is an excellent source of information on the state of the art in using biometrics (body feature) as a security access device. From retinal scans to typing error rates, this is a quick look at some of the available technologies. These will be increasingly used in health care settings as confidentiality concerns heighten.

Index

UMDNJ / Smith-Newark

3 3008 00581 9424

UMDNJ-SMITH LIBRARY
30 12TH AVENUE
NEWARK, N.J. 07103

DEMCO